NURSE JAN

Woman on a Pedestal

Ann Jasper R.N.

All rights reserved.
No part of; this book may be reproduced in any format
or in any medium without the written permission of Author, Ann Jasper

This is a work of fiction.
The characters, names, incidents, places, and dialogue are products
of the author's imagination, and not to be construed as real.

Copyright © 2012 Ann Jasper

All rights reserved.

ISBN: 1480086533
ISBN 13: 9781480086531

DEDICATION

MY FIRST NOVEL IS DEDICATED
TO MY VERY BEST FRIEND WHO
HAS SUPPORTED ME THROUGH THE
UPS AND DOWNS OF THIS
MOMENTOUS UNDERTAKING
I LOVE YOU CAROL HEGDAHL

ACKNOWLEDGEMENTS

MY SINCERE APPRECIATION IS EXTENDED TO
ALAYNE MATTHEWS
ANITA BOTT
KARL-ERIK BENNION, GRAPHIC DESIGNER
AND TO MY EDITOR
MARY E. BARNES, LITERARY COUCH, AGENT AND EDITOR

CHAPTER ONE
(1956)

DANGER AHEAD!

Janet Winston fought for her life! She had never known this kind of explosive terror, as if an atomic bomb had been ignited inside her gut while his strength smothered her in a cement shroud. He had grabbed her from behind as she tried to flee out the front door. Her heart pounded like the click, clack of the wheels on a train going 80 miles an hour she fought to spring free of his impregnable grip on her wrists. He held her from behind with his other hand over her mouth to stifle her screams. He caught the edge of the sofa with his foot, forcing it out from the wall as he pushed her in front of him, wedging her between the wall and the couch. He threw her down on the carpet like a garbage bag full of dirty rags to use and discard. She kicked and hit with her fists as he tore off her panties. She screeched as he whispered in her ear, "Come on, relax, I know you want it just as much as I do."

"No, I don't! Oh, please stop. Someone help me. please, don't!" He pushed his way into her, agonizing her very soul.

"I hate you. You're an animal!" she screamed. She felt as helpless as a tiny newborn, unable to stop him. Her brain moved into a fog of distraction from this ugly reality. As Jan sank into a mist of denial, she was unable to fully comprehend this vile act. Finally it was over. Jan opened her eyes to see him smile as he stood and zipped his trousers. "So beautiful," he whispered. "We will meet again, little one."

She lay limp, curled in a fetal position, murmuring, "No, no, never." He licked his lips as he made a quick exit out the front door. Jan was still frightened, feeling enormous physical and emotional pain. She knew she had to leave but was afraid he would be waiting for her outside to follow her to her apartment where he might force himself on her again. Slowly she pulled herself off the floor, hurting beyond repair. She just wanted to go home and die.

Jan grabbed what was left of her panties and purse and ran to her car. She zigzagged through the streets. Arriving home, she parked up the street instead of her designated spot in front; then ran up the stairs to her apartment, locking the door behind her. She stood at the door to catch her breath, imagining he might be lurking behind a door or in a closet. She turned on all the lights, opened every door, looked under the bed. Satisfied she was alone, she shoved a heavy chair to block her front door. Jan turned and sat on the edge of her bed. She rocked back and forth, her arms clutching her abdomen, moaning as her tears fell uncontrollably.

Finally she stripped off her dress and underclothes, threw them in the garbage and ran to the shower. She stood under the warm water scrubbing her skin raw until the water turned ice cold. With her pajamas and robe on, she lay wrapped in the covers like a camper enshrouded in a sleeping bag. She left all the lights on, afraid to be in the dark.

The evening had begun innocently enough in her college professor's home; a small crowd for drinks and conversation. When others excused themselves to leave, Jan found herself alone with her professor, his wife and his friend. The friend had deep ebony eyes, matching black hair and a wide mouth that remained straight when he smiled. "Will you stay for dinner, Miss Winston?" asked the professor.

They had started with some martinis, wine with dinner, followed by after-dinner drinks. She had politely sipped a glass of wine as she watched the alcohol twist their tongues and saturate their brains. They were no longer fun to be around; her hosts shocked her when they staggered from the living room to pour themselves into bed. When her hosts disappeared, he slid over close, getting way too friendly. Suddenly he grabbed her and landed a stinking kiss on her mouth! She wiggled free, excusing herself to use the bathroom. Once inside, she locked the door, rinsed her mouth out and made a plan. She would go into her professor's bedroom and ask for his help to escort her to her car. She quickly ran out of the bathroom to engage her plan. She knelt beside their bed, shaking him awake, begging for his help. His wavy dark brown hair covered his brown eyes as he turned away from her with slurred words, "Just leave. I'm sick!"

Almost overcome by his nasty breath, a mixture of alcohol and vomit, she begged, "Please, I'm afraid of him. Please help me."

"He's harmless. Just go home if you don't like him."

She could barely make out his words, feeling like a frightened child abandoned on a railroad track with the light barreling toward her. She went around to his wife, and there was flat out no response; Jan was not even sure she was alive. She made up her mind to make a run for it, and he was waiting at the door.

She couldn't fight him off. Her screams echoed throughout the room, falling on the waste pile of intoxication. Why, why, why? She wanted to erase the thoughts sprinkling around her mind like leftover fireworks and entangling her in a web of self incrimination. Had she been too friendly with him during dinner?

She hated Professor Buschke and his wife for ignoring her pleas for help. She couldn't even remember their friend's name. Should she tell someone? She knew no one would believe her. She was so ashamed, she wanted to die. She could never get married because she would have to tell him what happened. No decent man would want her. She hated herself.

Finally, sleep came; her brain was free to roam the darkness left inside. Her dreams cascaded with morbid visions of a useless, filthy, image of herself. She awoke, gasping for air. She sat up and screamed out loud, "I could be pregnant! Oh my God, no. What would I do? I know, I'd get an abortion. No one would have to know. Then I could just go on with my life like before." She threw her head back on the pillow. "NO," she screamed, "I could never do that; Please God, let me die!"

Jan stayed in bed all day Saturday, overcome with disdain for her body akin to a rotted out old car, left to rust, useless except to harbor small wiggly critters. Sunday she managed to eat some toast, read her textbook assignment and think how much she wanted to tell someone what had happened. She couldn't think of one person she could trust with such a morbid tale. She knew if she told her parents, her dad would want to kill him and her professor. By the end of the day she decided to go to work and school, lift her head high and keep her secret hidden deep within the private convolutions of her mind. If she ran into Professor Buschke in the hall she could hide or run the other way. Thank goodness she was no longer in his class. Jan never wanted to see his face or talk to him ever again. She couldn't believe this horrible experience had wedged its way into her comfortable routine of college and working in a hospital as a ward clerk in San Francisco.

Jan was determined to meet her goal of becoming a registered nurse; unless the unthinkable occurred. All she could do was wait for her next menstrual period. Once she passed that hurdle, she could go on with her plans and make believe none of this had ever happened.

CHAPTER TWO
(SAN FRANCISCO, CA 1957)

BEFUDDLED FEARS

Janet Winston, student nurse at Watkins Medical Center spun like a bumble bee caught in a glass jar on her hard dormitory mattress. At one point, she swung her feet over the side of the bed. The darkness of her room matched her dreary mood. She sat, holding her head in her hands, resting her elbows on her knees. Then she slowly stood to push her open window up all the way. The warm wet air smothered her as she visualized patients yelling and nurses scolding her. Jan's excitement about her first day working with real patients in the hospital was dampened by her emotions encircling her in a shroud of dread. Her nerves were over the edge. She let out a long sigh and climbed back into bed.

Eyes wide open, she tried to analyze her fear of interacting with real patients; fears that had led her into a murky pool of self-doubt. Her mind wandered to the phone call to her parents the previous evening,

"Hi, Mom. How are you and Dad doing?"

"We're fine, honey. is everything okay?"

"Yeah, I'm just real nervous tonight. That's all."

"What in the world are you nervous about, sweetheart?"

"Tomorrow's our first day working in the hospital, and I'm afraid I'll have a brain freeze and forget all I've learned in the last three months."

Her mother tried to stifle a giggle. "Well honey, isn't that what you've been working towards, being a real nurse?"

"Yes, of course, but I'm afraid I'll do something wrong!"

"Jan, you have worked in a hospital before. Did you do anything wrong then?"

"No, with the exception of the time I was holding a pint bottle of blood up for the nurse while she struggled with an IV standard and the cork popped out, covering me with blood."

"That wasn't your fault. The nurse hadn't put the cork in securely."

"I know, but I was just a ward clerk, and all I did with patients was deliver mail and do their paperwork. The only interaction was a cheery 'hello' and answering questions."

"Okay, honey, I understand. Listen, your dad is trying to wrestle me to the floor for the phone. I'll let you talk to him."

"Hi, Jan. How's my baby girl? Sounds like you're having some first day jitters."

"That's putting it mildly, Daddy!"

"I understand, honey. It's pretty normal to have those nerves tickling your tummy when you're about to embark on a new journey."

Jan felt a calmness sweep over her as she listened to her dad's voice.

He continued, "Now listen carefully. I guarantee as soon as daylight shines through your window, things will look better, and you will feel a surge of exhilaration knowing you're about to take a significant step towards your goal."

"Yeah, I guess so."

"Now, I have a sneaking hunch there is something else bothering you about tomorrow."

Jan stammered a bit, "Well, I think my biggest fear is that I have to face Miss Kingston tomorrow morning!"

"Oh, my goodness, darling. Tell me, does she have fangs and long claws?"

Jan laughed, "No Daddy."

"So she can't physically hurt you?"

Jan was still laughing, "No, but you have no idea how scary she is!"

"Is she as frightening as your mother?"

"Oh, now you're just being silly."

"No, I'm not. Your mother just came in from the kitchen armed with a meat cleaver, and that is scary!"

"Okay, you've made me feel better. Thank you, and tell Mom thanks, too. Others are lined up to use the dormitory phone. Love you. Bye."

She turned to apologize to other students who were lined up to make a call on the only phone available for their use.

Jan was thankful for the support of her parents. Her dad was moderate of height, muscular through his chest and arms, with the same iridescent blue eyes as Jan's. He had thinning hair and a smile that would gladden anyone's heart. Her mother revealed her emotions through her spirited brown eyes and a spicy smile. Jan had her mother's petite build and her firm determination to do what was right. Thinking of them, she felt a twinge of homesickness and missed their small town atmosphere where friends greeted her by name as they passed on the streets of home. The rolling hills were covered with shrubs and oak trees, especially the tree in their front yard she loved to climb when she was growing up. Then and now, everywhere she meandered hiking, riding a horse or her bike, she was surrounded by a breathtaking view of the snow capped mountains.

Being in the big city was only to accomplish her goal of becoming a registered nurse. If she could just get over her silly fears that were keeping her awake tonight; she wished she could understand her own anxieties. She instinctively knew there was a reason for these fears locked deep inside, but what was it? She knew it couldn't be the rape. Weeks had passed and Jan had never seen him again.

Suddenly Jan's alarm startled her out of her thoughts, and she jumped up, almost banging her knee on the chair of her desk. The room was so compact, if the metal desk and dresser were any smaller, she would think she was in a doll house. She threw on her robe while running down the hall to be the first in the bathroom. As she made it back to her room, there was an aura of excitement in the hall. "Today's the day," "We finally made it" and "I can hardly wait." She finally felt the exhilaration. Her father was right!

Janet started to put her long, naturally wavy, strawberry blonde hair into a ponytail when her door flew open and Mandy said, "Here, I'll do that," and twisted it into a perfect bun. "Hand me some hair pins, sweetness, and I'll be on my way."

"Thanks. Do you think they will notice if I crimp my eyelashes and put on a tiny bit of mascara?"

"I wouldn't try it if I were you. Remember the rules; we can only wear light-colored lipstick and absolutely no makeup or jewelry, with the exception of our nurse's wrist watch. We better hurry. I'll meet you in the cafeteria for breakfast," She spoke over her shoulder as she went for the door.

"Mandy, I'm not sure I can eat. I didn't sleep at all last night, and the thought of seeing the "Zombie" this morning makes me want to regurgitate!"

"Jan, are you practicing terminology on me again? You could easily say 'throw-up,' you know. I'll see you in the classroom."

"If my magic mirror tells me I'm the smartest, you will." She could hear Mandy laughing as she closed the door.

* * *

Jan and Mandy had hit it off from the first day in class. Mandy was the antithesis of Jan. Tall, big boned and husky, Mandy had a round face framed with dark, short hair and a wide mouth usually molded in a smile that crinkled her dark brown eyes. In class she was shy and usually sat in the back while Jan sat in front. That way, Jan could see only the instructor. If Jan saw the students looking at her, she would get a panic attack and not say anything. Mandy was younger, just out of high school. At twenty-one, Jan had a few years "growing up" experience behind her. Even with their differences, Jan and Mandy were fast becoming best friends, supporting each other in their individual weaknesses. Once, while walking together toward a full-length mirror, Mandy laughed saying, "I'm big enough to make two of you!"

"That's why I keep you around, so you can protect me from the Boogey Man!"

* * *

Jan sat on the edge of her bed to put on her white stockings, fastening them to a garter belt that fit snugly around her waist. She wiggled into her full length slip before carefully dressing in her uniform. First came her dress, made of heavy starched cotton- the same shade of blue as her eyes. The dress was accented with white cuffs and collar. Over this, she wore a stiffly starched white apron, tied in a bow at the back that accentuated her twenty-inch waist. The completed outfit was nearly ankle length; a perfect fit.

She studied herself in the square mirror over her dresser that reflected the light gray walls behind her. The more she looked at her image, the more Jan began to doubt herself, knowing she would soon face Miss Kingston. She turned away, slipped her feet into her white nursing shoes, and reached down to tie the laces. Jan glanced at her nurse's watch and flew out the door. Running through the courtyard and up the steps to the hospital entrance, she soaked in the humidity that promised another warm early October day. She couldn't wait for winter!

The class of students enrolled in the nursing program at Watkins Medical Center gathered in the classroom for a final briefing and inspection from Miss Kingston. As they walked in, Jan took Mandy's hand and gave it a quick squeeze before they paraded military style in front of their lead instructor. Three other instructors wearing expressionless faces, with their hands clasped behind their backs stood behind. Miss Kingston looked like a frozen ice sculpture in her starched white full-length uniform, buttoned at the neck with long cuffed sleeves to her wrists. She stood straight as a flagpole, with her black hair fastened in a tight bun at the back of her head. She wore no makeup over her pale skin, adding to her austere presence. Janet stood very still, afraid to move even one centimeter, hoping to blend in with the other students.

Miss Kingston stared at each class member, searching for flaws in hair, makeup or uniform. She fastened her dark eyes directly on Miss Winston. Jan felt a sense of terror envelop her, and wished she could transport herself into the pocket of her apron! Miss Kingston spoke, "Miss Winston, come here and stand in front of me."

CHAPTER THREE
FROM A TENT POLE TO SPAGHETTI

Jan's feet melted into the floor, making any effort to move impossible! She forced one foot in front of the other as she felt her cheeks turn a bright shade of red.

Miss Kingston put her icy hands on Jan's shoulders, sending a cool chill shimmering down her spine. Miss Kingston slowly turned Jan around in front of the students, "Class, take a good look at Miss Winston. This is the way everyone should look. Take a mental picture of your classmate and, remember, you will be graded on your appearance as well as your clinical nursing."

She turned her attention to Jan and in her usual stern voice said, "Come with me!"

As Jan followed, she caught Mandy giving her a look of "you poor thing." Jan took two steps for each of Miss Kingston's as they went into the hospital, rode up the elevator and stopped on the fourth floor. A sign on the opposite wall read "MEDICAL FLOOR."

Miss Kingston walked toward a smiling RN and said, "Mrs. Novak, this is Miss Winston, and she is reporting to you this morning. She then turned to Jan. Miss Winston, you will follow Mrs. Novak's instructions, and if either of you have a problem, just page Mrs. Jacob, the instructor assigned to this floor." Miss Kingston turned on her heel and quickly vanished down the hall.

The RN, probably in her early thirties, wore a small round nursing cap which looked like an upside down soup bowl huddling in tiny ruffles. Mrs. Novak had a rounded figure, was about the same height as Jan, and had a hint of mischief in her bright green eyes.

"Come on, I'll take you on a tour of the floor so you'll know where things are located."

When they returned to the nurses' station, she sat down with Jan. "I understand this is your first day assigned to patients in the hospital, correct?"

"Yes it is, but we've been practicing on each other in the classroom."

"That's great! Do you feel confident giving a bed bath?"

"I'm pretty sure I can."

She smiled as she explained, "You'll be doing a complete bed bath and bed change for Mr. Sorenson; he was involved in an automobile accident this morning and hasn't been cleaned up since his arrival in ER. I recommend that you read his chart before going to his room." She started to turn away, then added, "Oh, the patient's wife arrived a little bit ago and is in the room with him. Miss Winston, you need to politely ask her to wait down the hall while you clean him up. You know, we don't allow any visitors in the room while we are doing a procedure on a patient, right?"

"Yes, of course."

Miss Jan Winston made herself comfortable sitting at the nurses' station while she did a quick review of her patient's chart. She no sooner started reading when a doctor walked in. Jan quickly jumped up, moved away from the desk and sent her chair crashing to the floor! From her peripheral vision she saw that Mrs. Novak stood also, jumping from the sudden noise. Jan grabbed the chair, placed it upright, and attempted to recover from her embarrassment. Jan thought it was a stupid rule to stand up for a doctor when chairs were available, but it was a rule. Once he was gone, Jan sat down to resume her reading. Mr. Sorenson had been brought in by ambulance early in the morning after suffering severe head trauma in a head-on collision. He remained in a coma and would be watched closely for complications. She felt relieved knowing she wouldn't have to bathe a man who was awake.

She left the nurse's station, gathered her supplies, then walked to his room. Jan knocked, and then entered to see his young wife sitting by his side. Jan could see she'd been crying while he laid motionless, unaware of his surroundings.

"Good morning, Mrs. Sorenson. My name is Miss Winston, and I will be bathing your husband and changing his bed sheets. You can wait in the hall while I proceed."

Mrs. Sorenson stared at Jan without moving. "Did you understand what I said, Mrs. Sorenson?"

"Oh my, ah, yes of course. Ah, may I take a chair and sit in the hall by the door?"

"That would be fine, and I will hurry as fast as I can so you can come back."

Jan proceeded, washing off dirt that reeked with the odor of gasoline. She bathed as she had been taught, leaving his private parts for last. Had he been awake, she would have handed him the soapy washcloth and let him finish. She knew she was expected to complete the bath when a patient couldn't, so she dipped the washrag into the warm, sudsy water, wrapped it around his penis, and started washing. Mr. Sorenson began moaning as changes occurred to his anatomy. Jan's eyes widened and she felt like a piece of petrified wood as she stood staring at what she'd done. She threw the towel over it which didn't hide much as the towel resembled a tent. She worked in a fearful frenzy of being discovered through the rest of the procedure. Under her breath she whispered, oh please, don't let his wife open the door!

Trembling like a blender on full speed, she hurriedly gathered the dirty linens and wash basin. She practically knocked his wife off her chair as she flew out the door as if the room was possessed by a giant scorpion. In the utility room, Jan took a huge breath and muttered, "I can never tell another soul (well maybe Mandy) about this. It would travel the air currents back to Miss Kingston for sure, and she would twist me into the shape of a corkscrew."

Still calming herself, Jan started in the direction of the desk. She wanted to twirl away like a ballerina when she recognized her instructor talking to Mrs. Novak. Mrs. Jacob was much younger than Miss Kingston, of moderate height with an athletic build, sandy hair, cut short. She was usually pleasant and helpful but had a stern side as well.

Her teacher looked up and said, "Miss Winston, you need to take me back to the patient's room so I can check your work."

Jan stood still and silent as an iceberg, reluctant to return to the scene of her dastardly deed. Finally the words penetrated her brain, and Jan became aware that her instructor was standing next to her with a quizzical look.

"Miss Winston, did you hear me?"

"Yes," Jan said, mustering the courage to walk down the hall with Mrs. Jacob. Her instructor checked everything, including the modesty towel still over his groin area.

Mrs. Jacob made a comment as they returned to the desk. "At least I know that you used proper procedure Miss Winston, but in the future be sure you check the patient before you leave the room."

Jan felt the heat return to her face as she gave Mrs. Jacob a weak smile and shook her head yes. "Just answer lights, then help pass lunch trays. Mrs. Novak will assign you a patient to feed." her instructor said as she left the station.

It was fun answering lights; most of the requests were for pain pills, refill water pitchers or to help patients use the bedpan.

By the time lunch trays arrived, Jan had nearly forgotten her little episode of the morning.

She was assigned to feed a seventeen-year-old, brain injured male patient. Jan felt her heart pound as she opened the door to his room.

"Hi, I'm Miss Winston and - - -" He looked terribly uncomfortable, curled up like a deformed pretzel with his head up against the side rails. His body was like the skeleton in anatomy lab with a thin layer of tissue paper covering his bones. She brought him up to a comfortable position, braced him with pillows, and washed some saliva off his face before serving lunch. He couldn't speak, yet he never took his expressive brown eyes off of her as she fed him bites of spaghetti, a roll and some applesauce. Jan knew she needed to talk to him and treat him like he was normal, but what could she say?

"It's a warm day out; would you like another spoonful of applesauce?" She glanced around his room. "You have a lot of nice cards; you must have many friends." She could feel the warmth of his soul answering without sounds of his mouth.

"I'll bet you don't like someone stuffing food in your mouth, but maybe someday you'll be able to do it yourself. In the meantime, you're going to have to put up with me, and you'll have to admit I shovel pretty well."

When he finished, Jan washed his face and cleaned up around him, feeling reluctant to leave him alone again. "I'll be back to see you again. Maybe we can go out on a dinner date next time." His eyes answered her with the sound of silent laughter. Jan walked out of his room feeling good about her choice to be a nurse.

She had just enough time to grab some lunch and hurry back to work until two when she would attend a nursing class.

Jan went back to answering lights. She saw one go on over a door and flew out of the nurse's station. As she rushed down the hall her starched uniform and white apron made a "shushing" sound while her legs ran like a jet propelled lawn mower. She felt a sense of excitement as she cautiously opened the door and asked, "Can I help you?"

All Jan could see were strings of spaghetti tinged with red sauce hanging from the metal side rails. A patient was hanging over the side rail. Perspiration was soaking her blond curls causing them to stick to her forehead. She spoke in a raspy voice, "Oh, I'm so sick!" She threw up again. Jan jumped back wondering how much spaghetti could fit in one's stomach.

She looked at the floor between her and the patient's bed and knew her feet would go right out from under her if she stepped to her bedside. Grabbing her wash basin, she reached over to hand it to the patient, "Use this if you feel sick again. I'm going out to get supplies and I'll be right back."

"Oh, hurry please. I'm so very sick. Bring me something to stop this, please!"

"I'll tell the nurse, okay?" Jan blurted as she ran out the door.

As Jan walked quickly past the nurses' station, she slowed to report, "Mrs. Novak, the patient in room 436, has regurgitated all over the place. she needs something STAT! As Jan acquired her supplies, the thought occurred to her that cleaning up disgusting messes was not part of the bargain for becoming a nurse. It made her wonder if she was just as crazy as those men who talked about flying around in outer space!

After spending an hour mopping the floor, cleaning the patient, changing her bed and watching the RN give her an injection for her nausea (wondering if she could ever do that) Jan continued to monitor the call lights until class.

Just ten minutes before time to report to the classroom, the "spaghetti patient" rang her light again. Jan stood transfixed, knowing she couldn't face that a second time. She eased her gaze in the opposite direction hoping someone else would answer the light.

Mrs. Novak looked up from her charting, "Miss Winston, there's a light on."

She moved considerably slower towards the room this time. With great trepidation, Jan reluctantly pushed the door open, and the patient sat up in bed and smiled at Jan like a bouncing clown on a penny arcade. "You left before I could say thank you. You did such a good job, and you made me feel much better. You're going to be a great nurse!"

"Thank you. Is there anything else I can do for you?"

"No, I'm fine now. Thanks for coming back."

Miss Jan Winston Student Nurse knew she could do anything she put her mind to. She had climbed a huge boulder and was standing on top.

* * *

The following day, as the nursing students rode back from the college campus on the bus provided by the hospital, Edna spoke up, "Hey everybody, we are going to have a quick meeting tonight at the Pizza Parlor to discuss the skit we have to perform for the senior class in December. We need to make some major plans since December is right around the corner. She turned towards Jan. "Miss Winston, when we had our closed vote the other day, the freshman class unanimously chose you to play the leading role. So we will build the skit to fit the character you want to play. Put your brain on full-speed ahead and tell us after dinner."

"I don't want to be in the skit, let alone the lead! Please get someone else!" Edna laughed, thinking Jan was playing coy. "Sorry, it's set in stone, no backing out now!"

Jan slumped down in her seat, feeling her world implode around her. She'd been very successful hiding her secret from everyone. They had no idea she suffered from crippling panic attacks when she had to speak in front of people. She was keenly aware her classmates looked up to her, probably because she was the oldest and now her secret would be revealed and she'd take a nose dive off her pedestal.

As they walked upstairs, Jan asked Mandy, "Will you come in my room a minute?"

As they walked in, Mandy looked at her friend. "Why so gloomy all of a sudden?"

"Oh, Mandy I'm a big fat fraud! Everyone looks up to me, but I have a deep dark secret I have hidden from everyone, including you!"

Mandy quickly sat in the chair, slapping her forehead. "What are you, a serial killer who's lost a whole lot of weight?"

"Mandy, I'm serious. Stop being funny!"

"Okay, I'm sorry; you're probably not a serial killer, but you most certainly have become a skinny fraud."

Jan couldn't help but chuckle. "Okay, you got me there. Now I really need to tell you my problem."

"I'm listening."

"I suffer from horrible panic attacks when I get up in front of a crowd and have to speak. I start trembling all over, my heart beats out of my chest and I can't remember what I'm supposed to say! I act just like the comedian Don Knotts, but it's for real."

"Jan, it's okay. Most of us suffer from the same thing. But, hey, you could put it into the skit if you played his part. Everyone knows his act and the whole skit can be worked around your panic attack and not a soul will know it's real."

"You're right. I think I could do it; I'll just copy him when he gets all nervous, shaking and stammering."

* * *

At the pizza parlor as they sat waiting for their pizza, a couple of Jan's classmates whispered in her ear, "Why don't you buy a pitcher of beer and we'll all share?" They slid some money in front of her.

"Absolutely not!" Jan answered, sliding the money back. "I'm the only one of legal age to buy alcohol, so I'd be held liable for breaking the law."

"Well, excuse me for asking!" Cindy, a perky little blonde, walked away to sit at another table, then glared at Jan as if she was an infidel of the worst kind.

Mandy calmly said, "Jan just forget it; someday Cindy will grow up. Besides, if you did what she wanted, I can see the headlines, "Student Nurse Arrested for Procuring Alcohol for Minors!"

"Hmm, would you visit me in jail?"

"Heck no. I'm not going to be seen associating with a hardened criminal!" said Mandy. Everyone at the table laughed. After dinner Jan made her suggestion. Edna looked at her while laughing hysterically. "That's a great idea. We can work a super skit around it! Okay girls, let's write a play around Miss Jan Knotts."

CHAPTER FOUR

NO DATING FOR THIS NURSE

As Jan and her group of student nurses were on their way to class, one of her classmates ran into an old friend from her hometown. Jan was curious as the other girls stopped and turned to look at him. Jan caught him gazing at her with his deep, dark brown eyes. As Sherry was introducing everyone, Jan felt her knees buckle as if she'd been hit from behind by a baseball bat. She was embarrassed as her eyes fixed on him like they'd been super glued. He returned her stare. Electric shocks tingled through Jan's body when Sherry spoke. "Jan, I'd like you to meet Allen Morris."

He came forward and took her hand, not letting go like he had the others. "Did you say Jan? Is that short for Janet?"

She could only shake her head as she croaked, "Yes."

"What do you like to be called, Jan or Janet?"

Jan took in his incredibly good looks while his dark eyes continued to pierce right to her soul. He had brown hair, worn in a crew cut, with dark eyebrows that made a perfect outline over his eyes. His skin was smooth, and he sported a golden tan. He was freshly shaved and had slight outlines on both sides of his mouth that indicated he was accustomed to smiling.

"I prefer Jan, Jan Winston."

Still holding her hand, he said, "Jan, I have never seen such incredibly beautiful blue eyes in my entire life." She started to say thank you when the bell rang, and they separated to run to their classes.

With her thoughts racing, Jan barely listened to the teacher. Her encounter was unlike anything she had experienced before. She tried desperately to take notes, while her thoughts wandered to the commitment she had made to focus solely on her education. She didn't need the distractions of dating. She needed to put a lid on these feelings as you would put a lid on a fry pan spitting hot oil on the stove.

Finally the bell rang. She entered the hall, and there he was again, slouching against the wall with one foot bent under him. His eyes greeted her with a huge grin. He walked over, then matched his step with hers. "What room are you headed to?" Allen asked.

She whispered, "Room 220 upstairs."

He looked at her and spoke with a smile that reached out and encircled her heart. "That's the same direction I'm going. I'll walk you to your room." He leaned over, taking her books and grasped them under his muscular arm.

She felt numb from her waist down, as she softly drifted up the stairs. Jan came to her room and stopped. She reached for her books. Before he handed them to her, he asked, "May I give you a ride home?"

She stammered, "We r-ride a bus back to the nurse's dormitory."

He continued to look down at her and answered, "Fine, we can stop and let the bus driver know. Where's your last class?"

"Room 156 in 'B' Building."

"I'll pick you up outside the door. See you then."

Jan watched Allen's lean body move easily between other students until he disappeared. *Wow.*

* * *

As her last class ended, the gyro movement inside her torso returned. It felt like a million little people doing a tap dance inside her belly. She began talking to herself saying, Maybe he won't even be there. Maybe he doesn't want to date a nurse. Why am I thinking of dating? Then her thoughts went back to her commitment. If he isn't there, I'll be off the hook. I can forget I ever saw him and continue with my studies.

Jan took her time walking out the door, and right there, standing against the wall, was Allen with a big smile on his face. He walked over and took her books. He brushed against Jan's hand as her breath lodged in the middle of her throat.

Just as he promised, they walked to the bus. "Hey, Bill, I won't be riding the bus back." Jan said to the bus driver. He leaned forward and took a good look at Allen. "He looks safe enough, thanks for telling me."

The other students drooled all over the windows as Jan and Allen walked away.

He took her hand in his and guided her to the parking lot. They walked up to a gray Volkswagen Bug, and he opened the passenger door for her. The seats were only separated by a long handled gear shift. There was no automatic shift. Jan stared straight ahead, afraid he would catch her looking at him. Her hands were shaking so badly, she held them tightly together in her lap.

Allen broke the ice as he pulled out of the parking lot. "So, how do you like being a nurse?"

"I love it, and I'm determined to stay centered on my education until I graduate in two- and-a-half years."

He glanced at her and asked, "Does that mean you're not allowed to date?"

"Pretty much, yes."

He laughed softly and said, "How about lunch and a ride to campus? Would that fit into your agenda?"

Jan couldn't help but chuckle as she answered, "That would be just fine."

Allen grinned from ear to ear. With no effort to hide his excitement he exclaimed, "Great! Now how about a quick dinner tonight, and I will take you right back to your dorm so you can study?"

Surprised, she heard herself answering, "Okay. I do have to eat, as long as I can study tonight."

He turned the bug in another direction and drove to a pizza parlor named the "Zombie Zulu Hut."

As Allen shut off the engine, Jan asked, "How did you find a place with such a funny name?"

"Don't make fun of it. The pizza's the best in town." said Allen. He jumped out and ran around the car to open her door. When he reached down to take her hand, their eyes met and Jan felt like she was made of wax, exposed to a hot flame.

Inside the cafe, they ordered Jan's favorite, mushroom and sausage, before sitting in a booth. The decorations inside matched the name. It was like sitting in the middle of the jungle, surrounded with shrunken heads, spears and native paraphernalia. She started to laugh. "Are you sure they serve pizza here? I expect them to stuff us in a boiling caldron at any minute."

"No, they only do that if they run out of sausage." Allen quipped. They both laughed. Allen cocked his head to the side, with a quizzical look. "How long have you been going to college?"

"Ever since I graduated from high school."

"Wow, you must be all of nineteen then?"

"No, I spent a few years at another college getting my prerequisites and working as a ward clerk in a hospital. I'm twenty-one."

"Whew, that's a relief. For a minute I thought I was robbing the cradle."

"Why? How old are you?"

"Jan, I returned a year ago after four years in the United States Air Force, stationed on Okinawa during the Korean Conflict. I turned twenty-five a couple of weeks ago. And I'm determined to accomplish my goal of becoming a dentist."

They found they had a lot in common; both enjoyed movies, camping, hiking and riding horses. Time flew and it wasn't long before Jan had to get back to study before curfew. They agreed that he would pick her up for lunch and a ride to school the day after next. He drove her to the dorm, and as they walked hand in hand to the front door, he leaned over to give her a quick kiss on the cheek. Then he ran back to his car. Jan watched as he drove out of sight.

Many of the girls, including their "House Mom" were studying in the common room. They were filled with questions and comments about Allen. She answered a few questions before she turned and ran up the stairs to her room. As she entered her dorm room, Mandy was already busy studying. "Well, Miss Cinderella, anything new in your life, or is that a forbidden subject?"

"Oh, Mandy, I can't believe this happened to me. I told myself I would never date while I was in nurses training. Now look at me. I'm a blubbering idiot over this man!"

Mandy chuckled, "Never say never my dear friend."

"I'm reeling in disbelief. Has this really happened, or will I wake up any minute?"

"Well, right now you had better wake up, take off your princess crown, and get to studying, or your prince will turn into a pumpkin."

That night Jan could hardly sleep. While she lay there in the dark, she could not help feeling she had met her future.

CHAPTER FIVE
MAGGOTS AND LEECHES, OH NO!

While on the medical wing, Jan was assigned to Mrs. Nowakowski, an elderly female brought to the hospital by her daughter, Sarah. Sarah had moved her mother into her home when her mother suffered a stroke and could no longer live alone. Not having any medical knowledge, Sarah allowed her mother to stay seated in her chair for hours at a time. As a result, she developed a very large decubitus ulcer or bed sore. Jan admitted Mrs. Nowakowski from the emergency room and turned to read the doctor's orders from her chart: "Three ounce jar of maggots, Hydrogen Peroxide, 3 packages of sterile gauze, and tape."

Jan read the order three times and then paged Mrs. Jacob. When her instructor arrived Jan promptly asked, "What are maggots?"

Her instructor laughed, "Little creatures that you are going to become very familiar with."

Jan frowned, "What kind of little creatures?"

"They are tiny little larvae used to remove dead and infected tissue from a wound such as the type your patient has. They are harmless except to the bacteria eating away the tissue and preventing normal healing."

Jan cringed. "Do I have to touch them?"

"Yes, but only with gloves on. Now go to the pharmacy and pick them up, then gather the other supplies, and I will meet you in the room to take a look at her ulcer."

Jan quickly returned from the pharmacy. Mrs. Nowakowski was in bed, lying on her side. She was awake and had some difficulty speaking as a result of her stroke. She seemed very lethargic and just wanted to rest.

Mrs. Jacob turned down the covers to reveal a large, five-inch diameter, deep ulcer at the base of her spine. The ulcer was filled with purulent material. Jan stepped back in horror, knowing she dared not say a word in front of the patient.

Mrs. Jacob asked, "Miss Winston, do you remember how a decubitus forms?"

Jan answered, "When a person becomes sedentary. If they remain in one position for hours, the pressure on the skin prevents the blood flow. This in turn keeps the cells from receiving nourishment, so they eventually die, which breaks down the tissue. Infection sets in and becomes what is commonly known as a bed sore."

"Very good. Do you have any questions?"

Jan, still reeling from what she saw, whispered, "Is she in pain?"

"Surprisingly, no. Oh, there may be some discomfort deep inside, but she feels very little pain."

Just then the doctor strolled in, looking directly at Jan. "Are you ready?" he asked her.

"Yes, doctor."

Gloves were applied, and the doctor cleansed the wound. Jan picked up the glass jar and removed the lid as the doctor opened his hand for her to shake the critters in. He placed them inside the ulcer, and they eagerly involved themselves in their gourmet dinner. Mrs. Nowakowski continued to sleep, unaware of her new roommates. Fascinated, Jan watched what was taking place.

Then Mrs. Jacob dropped the bomb. "I'm glad you're watching so closely, Miss Winston, because you will be doing the treatment tomorrow."

Jan swallowed hard, looking down at the almost empty jar and whimpered, "Will you be here to help me?"

Mrs. Jacob nodded. "I wouldn't think of letting you do this on your own. Not yet anyway."

Jan's first question the next day was, "What do I do with the old maggots?"

Mrs. Jacob had a twinkle in her eye as she replied, "Gather up what's left of them in the gauze bandage. Now clean the area and apply the fresh maggots to the wound."

Jan did as she was told even though she could feel them wiggling in her gloved hand. Once it was over, Jan turned to her instructor with a big sigh. "That wasn't too awfully bad, now that it's over."

"Good. you'll be doing it again tomorrow and I will also teach you how to debride the ulcer."

In the coming weeks, this procedure was taught during a lesson in Jan's nursing class. They were also taught about the use of leeches in reducing edema and in treating external hemorrhoids. Jan couldn't help but wonder when she would come face to face with a leech. *Ugh!*

A couple of weeks later, her wish was granted. An elderly male patient in renal failure was placed under her care. Mr. Flanders had severe edema over his entire body, so severe his lower extremities were dripping with fluid! It looked like he had just stepped out of the shower. His abdomen was so distended; it reminded Jan of an over-sized weather balloon ready to burst. Jan placed towels under his legs to protect the sheets.

One of the RN's walked into the room, carrying a large glass container of leeches and a catheterization tray. "Mr. Flanders, I'm going to assist Miss Winston in your care today. The doctor has ordered us to insert a catheter into your bladder to remove some of the fluid. We are also going to place these leeches on your legs to help draw the excess fluid out of your body."

"What are you going to do first?"

"We'll catheterize you first. Have you had this procedure before, Mr. Flanders?"

"Yes, many times. I'm used to it."

"Miss Winston, have you catheterized a patient before?"

"Yes, female patients and I've observed a male."

"Okay, put on the sterile gloves, and I'll walk you through it."

The RN gave excellent instructions and Jan was able to place it properly. It was amazing how much fluid gushed out. Jan now felt confident in doing this procedure by herself.

Mr. Flanders commented, "You're as good as the doctor."

"Thank you."

The RN said, "We're now going to place the leeches."

Mr. Flanders was shaking with apprehension as he asked, "Are they going to bite me?"

"No, they should actually relieve some of the discomfort you're experiencing at the moment. Do you like licorice, Mr. Flanders?" the nurse asked.

"Yes, I love licorice!"

"Well, as you can see, they look similar to a shiny piece of licorice. They're very sluggish in their movements acting like a suction cup, drinking in the fluid. Miss Winston and I will place these."

"Are you sure it won't be painful?"

"Not at all Mr. Flanders. Like I said, they will make you feel better."

"Okay, as long as I will feel better, go ahead."

Jan experienced the use of these strange creatures many times while serving as a student nurse. It never failed to amaze her how well they did their assigned jobs.

CHAPTER SIX
(December - 1957)

PANIC TO PICKLED

While walking back to their rooms following a nursing class, the other students reminded Jan, that they had their big performance tomorrow night. She knew she couldn't avoid this commitment, but every time they rehearsed, her panic attacks skyrocketed past Mars! How could she possibly go through with this?

Jan stood outside the door to the classroom wearing white pants and a blouse covered by an oversized lab coat. A surgical hat sat lopsided on her head. She wore oversized horn rimmed glasses and gobs of red lipstick and blush. A mask, surgical gloves and a stethoscope stuck haphazardly out of the coat pockets. She began to hyperventilate as her heart took off on a flight around the world. She was shaking like leaves fluttering off trees in a high wind. Jan was about to bolt and run when the door opened and Mandy gave her opening line, "Oh look, our new instructor, Miss Knotts has arrived."

Jan walked in, giving the impression that she was scared to death and she was. She gawked at the audience, as they laughed hysterically. As the laughter subsided, Jan turned toward her "students" and fumbled for notes inside her pocket. Her "sterile" gloves landed on the floor. Accidentally stepping on the gloves, Jan reached down for them saying, "Humph, oh well, these are still good enough to use on Miss Kingston's surgery." She stuffed the notes back in her pocket.

The line that received the biggest applause and laughter was when she picked up a bedpan and in a loud voice said, "Now class, you must carefully observe this, it is a glorified portable potty." She lifted it and looked inside. "What is this? My goodness, it looks like poop!" Getting her nose very close, she took a sniff. "It definitely smells like poop!" Reaching inside the bedpan, Jan poked the brown blob with the end of her finger, took a lick and exclaimed, "It definitely tastes like poop! Mrs. Jacob, have you been using my personal bedpan again?"

It took awhile for the laughter to subside, giving her time to swallow the peanut butter, rub her tummy and give a loud sigh. Jan slowly became aware that her own anxiety was decreasing and she was actually acting the part. The skit went well, judging by the amount of laughter, she enjoyed the moment as her initial panic subsided. The compliments that followed showed how well she played the part. Mandy said she was born to be an actress. Even Miss Kingston said it was the best skit she'd ever seen. Only Mandy knew the relief Jan felt.

When they returned to their rooms, Mandy threw her arms around Jan. "I knew you could do it. You were fantastic!"

"I can't believe it, Mandy. My panic flew out the window about half way through."

Mandy handed her a little plastic nurse on a pedestal. "See, you're still on your pedestal." Jan cried and they hugged again.

* * *

(Early March, 1958)

Sunday morning Jan stood in front of the mirror and decided to change to yet another outfit. She was anxious, knowing she would be spending the whole day with Allen. They had never been together more than an hour or so at a time. As she slipped into a poodle skirt worn with a crinoline slip, she rehearsed in her mind what Allen had said. "Be sure and dress comfortable for a long ride." From her upstairs window she could see the cars turning into the main drive of the hospital. Just then, she spotted his little Volkswagen. The sun bounced off his windshield promising the possibility of an early spring. She threw her skirt and slip on the bed and jumped into Levis. She let out a squeal, grabbed her purse and a jacket, and ran down the stairs to the front door. As he rang the doorbell, she felt those little people return to her stomach doing their dance routine. He greeted her with a hug and walked her to the car and opened the door.

They were quiet as he maneuvered his car around traffic. Allen spoke first. "You've never told me how your skit went for the senior nurses back in December?"

"Goodness, I'd almost forgotten all about it. Well, everyone said they really liked it, and Miss Kingston actually said it was the best ever!"

"Well of course, you were the star, Jan." He paused, taking out a stick of gum, and chewed until it was soft. "So when did you realize you wanted to pursue a nursing career?"

"Actually, I had always wanted to be an actress, but my brother-in-law set me straight when I was nearing graduation from high school. That's when I decided to take some college prep courses and work in a hospital environment to see if I liked it."

"That's funny, I always figured I'd take over my folks cattle ranch until I went to our local dentist with a toothache, right after I was discharged. He talked to me for an hour about the shortage of dentists. Then he let me hang around the office observing, and I decided I wanted to do it."

"People can have a powerful influence on our lives, can't they?"

"Yes, some for good and some bad." He said with a touch of sarcasm.

"Do you care to elaborate on that?"

"No, not now. Maybe later."

Jan wondered what that was all about when she realized they were in the countryside, heading up into the hills. They continued to talk about their chosen careers and what they each wanted to accomplish in life as they covered many miles. Jan asked, "Okay, are you going to tell me where we are going, or does that remain a secret also?"

His eyes sparkled as he turned to her and asked, "Do you really want to know?"

"Well of course I do, silly."

She felt herself melt as Allen looked at her with his irresistible smile and answered, "Guess what?"

"What?" She giggled.

"The only way I will tell you is if you let me give you a great big kiss right now."

Jan felt her nerves bolt together in a supercharged twang. She laughed, "You're driving a car; you can't give me a kiss."

His brown eyes pierced hers. "So, if I weren't driving a car, you would let me?"

Before she could take another breath to answer, he pulled off the road, shut off the car, jumped out, and ran around to her side. When he reached her door, he opened it, took her hand gently and pulled her up in front of him. He looked at Jan as she glimpsed the sun turning his brown hair golden. Their eyes spoke a language of their own as he wrapped his arms around her. They kissed with such a reverence, it overwhelmed her. He drew back, looking at her for a few seconds, then he dropped his head down for a more fervent kiss.

Jan was sure her system had shut down as she lost all her strength. They gently held on to each other, with her head on his arm as he said, "What have you done to me, Miss Winston? I can't stop thinking about you. I have never met anyone like you before; you're everything I ever wanted in a woman."

Just then, someone laid on their horn as they passed, and Allen said, "I guess we'd better be on our way, Pumpkin." Jan melted as she slid into the seat. They drove off in silence, each lost in the reverie of their own thoughts. Finally Allen spoke. "Jan, I have traveled all over the world in the Air Force, searching for the kind of woman I would want to be with for the rest of my life, and she was right here in my own backyard."

Jan was utterly speechless. She sat in the seat next to him, completely drained of energy. She could not get over the feel of his strong arms around her and his lips against hers. She had no idea where he was taking her, but she knew she wanted to take this journey with him.

Coming to her senses, she said, "You promised you would tell me where we're going if I let you kiss me."

He laughed and answered, "Wow, I almost forgot! Look up in those hills way ahead and you can see our destination."

"Okay, but I still don't know what is up there."

"It's my hometown, where I was born and raised."

They began an ascent, winding around foothills. After crossing a bridge, they made a sweeping turn into a country town lined with small shops mingled with well-preserved buildings from a prior century. A few people waved at Allen as he turned off the main street and continued on a small rural road that wound around the hills with ranches dotting the countryside. Suddenly, a thought occurred to her. "Are you taking me to meet your family?"

"Yes, I can't wait for my mom to meet you."

Jan froze, hoping she would awaken from this dream. She didn't feel ready to meet anyone. Her inclination was to grab the wheel, spin it into a U-turn and tell Allen to take her home. Instead she asked, "Do we have to see your family?"

"Yes, Pumpkin, probably only my mom."

She looked at the expression on his face and knew she had to see this through. Allen pulled off the road onto a narrow lane, surrounded on both sides with green pastures and dotted with cows and horses. They turned a corner, and way ahead she could see a large cream-colored, two-story house surrounded by landscaping and stately trees that took her breath away. The lane ended at the entrance of a circular driveway. They pulled up in front of the house and parked. Allen jumped out, pulling her into another quick embrace and said, "Let's go meet my mom."

They walked up the wide staircase and across a porch that appeared to go around the entire house. The door opened and there stood a petite lady with dark hair, cut short, with natural waves framing her face. She smiled with motherly love that focused on her son. Allen took her in his arms, kissed her and said, "Mom, I would like you to meet Jan Winston. Jan, this is my mom, Carmela."

Jan immediately knew where Allen got his brown eyes. His mother turned and gave Jan a hug and said, "Welcome to our home. Come with me into the kitchen so we can visit while I fix a meal for you." She took Jan by the hand and led her into the spacious and welcoming house.

Jan felt comfortable around Carmela. The house, with a homey and inviting atmosphere, made Jan want to curl up like a contended kitty cat. The kitchen surrounded her with the aromas of garlic, basil and cinnamon. It was adorned with yellow curtains and rooster-decorated walls and shelves. She and Jan talked as if they'd known each other for years.

Allen cleared his throat and said, "I think I'll look around outside." At the same time the back door slammed and a gruff voice hollered, "Has that no good son of ours arrived yet?" Jan hoped Allen's father was kidding when he came around the corner and gave his son a bear hug from behind that seemed more like a death grip than a welcome hug. His father barely acknowledged her as she was introduced. Jan had a strange feeling about him.

They stayed for a meal. Jan was deeply concerned with the degrading behavior of Allen's father, as he crawled into a bottle of whiskey and drowned. He was abrasive, negative and exhibited the language of the town drunk. Jan could see visible signs of embarrassment in Allen and his mother. She was grateful when Allen said they should leave after their meal and his mother encouraged their abrupt departure.

They began the drive home. Jan was quiet, reflecting on the events of the day. Allen was unusually quiet as well.

Finally, Jan blurted out, "I really liked your mother, and the meal was delicious."

Allen didn't answer. He remained quiet for a few minutes and chewed on his gum like a cow chewing on her cud. He turned on another road, mumbling, "I'm taking a short cut." When they had gone a couple of miles, he turned off and opened a gate where a sign was posted "DO NOT ENTER." He then started up a steep hill on a dirt road. He was so quiet that Jan wasn't sure how to take his strange behavior.

They crested the top, stopping where the road ended at a sign "PRIVATE PROPERTY, NO TRESPASSING." In silence he opened her door, took her hand and walked over to the edge. She gasped as she looked down at the sudden drop off below her feet.

CHAPTER SEVEN

HIS FATHER'S SHAME

Jan felt a pang of fear as she looked down at what seemed an endless drop-off below her feet! She had never felt anything but total trust from this man before this moment, which confused her sense of judgment. She instinctively knew she needed to separate Allen from his father and put the two men in separate boxes. Close the one with his father in it and throw it over the cliff as she opened Allen's box.

He dropped her hand and slid his arm around her waist, "This is my favorite view in the whole world."

Her worry flew off on the crest of a wind gust. She took in the panorama of the foothills that ended with a dramatic backdrop of snow capped mountains. The clear blue sky laced with wisps of brush stroked clouds seemed too perfect to be real.

Her curiosity got the better of her. "It's a breathtaking view, but aren't we trespassing on someone's property?"

"It's okay, I know the owner."

They stood there with their arms around each other, drinking in the view; then he turned her toward him, reaching down to kiss her once again. It was a sweet and tender kiss, filled with emotion.

A soft breeze blew Jan's hair, and he gently reached down to touch it, whispering, "You are so beautiful." Jan again felt secure and warm in his arms as he kissed her. They walked hand in hand back to the car. Instead of starting the car, he turned toward her and spoke in an emotional tone. "I owe you an explanation regarding my father."

Jan wasn't sure she wanted to open the box she had watched disappear at the bottom of the canyon. She wanted to say, *Why do you and your mom put up with his rotten attitude?* But she kept her thoughts to herself and turned to face him, she said "Sure, go ahead."

Glancing at Jan and seeing her look of expectancy, Allen cleared his throat and began. "My dad was a wonderful father, gentle and kind as I grew up. He took me fishing. We played ball together and he was always there for me. He taught me to be honest, to enjoy life, and to respect a woman's virtue. He treated my mother with love, setting an example for me to follow. I loved my father deeply and tried to pattern my life after his."

Allen hesitated, watching Jan's reaction.

"Tell me more, Allen." *How can he be talking about the man I just met?*

"When I was thirteen, my dad volunteered as a Deputy Sheriff for the county. My dad went through the training and received his uniform. We were very proud of him and enjoyed hearing about his experiences. After two years on the force he answered a call for an armed robbery. He was on patrol and the first on the scene. He saw a teenager running away from the house and ordered him to stop. He had to chase him on foot until the kid was cornered by a high fence. He saw him pull a gun out of his pocket. My dad told him to put down his weapon or he would shoot. Instead the kid raised the weapon directly toward my dad. He had no choice but to shoot. He aimed for his leg to drop him, and apparently the bullet hit his femoral artery. The teenager bled to death in my dad's arms. When help arrived, my dad reached down to pick up the teenager's gun for evidence. To his absolute horror, he realized the gun was a toy."

"Even though he was cleared of any wrong doing, Dad has never been the same. He took to staying up late, drinking with his buddies at the local bar and sunk into a deep depression. My mom and I tried everything to change his sour moods but nothing helped. It became so bad, when I turned nineteen I felt prompted to join the military just to get away. I have grieved for the loss of my father as I once knew him and longed to have him back as he was before."

Allen was filled with emotion while he talked, and Jan felt the tears rise to her eyes. She knew there was nothing she could do but offer her emotional support and understanding. "I'm so sorry you've gone through so much."

He continued, "I had hoped to see a change when I returned home from overseas. If anything, his attitude towards my mom had worsened. I couldn't stand anymore and confronted my dad; he turned physically abusive! I could have dropped him in his tracks, but my military training wasn't designed to harm my father. Instead I just turned my back, packed my things and left. I begged my mother to go with me but she could only cry and say, "I can't leave my home!"

"Today was the first time I've seen him since I left a year ago. I've been in constant contact with my mother, and she remains firm in her conviction that maybe someday he will change. After today, I've pretty much given up hope."

"I can understand why you feel that way. On the other hand, I can relate to your mom believing he may change. It's a woman thing."

He smiled as he said, "I'm sorry I used you as a buffer. What I really wanted to do was have a reason to spend the day with you. He grinned wider. I may be pushing my luck but in my day dreams I shrink to pocket size so I can stay close to you all the time. I will, however, remain committed to both of us reaching our goals."

Before Jan could answer, he said, "You have captured my heart little lady and I will abide by any rules of behavior that you choose so I can stay in your life." He let out a laugh as they started winding their way down the hill to head home, and said, "Give me a list, Pumpkin."

Jan reeled with emotion. While she sat and pondered all that had been said, she began to mentally make a list. She turned to look at him, felt her stomach do another flip-flop and said, "Okay, first nothing can stop me from becoming an RN; for now that has to be my priority. Second, total honesty in our relationship; and third, no sex before marriage." She took a quick glance to see how he had reacted to that last one and found him smiling back at her. *Hum, she wondered, was he smiling because he approved or thought he could talk her out of it?*

He continued to grin he said, "Okay, I can live with all of that. Now can we assume that we will not date anyone else?"

Mildly surprised, Jan answered, "Given the fact that I was determined not to date at all, I would say that's a yes."

Allen almost ran off the road as he exclaimed, "Janet Winston, you've made my day!"

As they pulled up in front of the nurse's dormitory, he parked, turned off the engine but did not get out of the car. Instead, he turned towards her and said, "Open the glove compartment, Jan and take out the small box you will find there."

Jan felt her heart take a magic leap as she took out a small, square box. She opened it, and her mouth flew open as she saw a lovely solitaire cultured pearl ring, set in white gold. She couldn't think of a thing to say as she looked at Allen as if to say, *"For me?"*

It was like he knew her thoughts as he said, "Pumpkin, take it out and try it on." He watched expectantly as she slipped it on her ring finger. She could see that it fit her perfectly.

Jan looked at him and asked, "How did you know my size?"

He said, "You will never believe this, but I will tell you anyway. When I was in Hong Kong a few years ago, I saw that ring and knew that I wanted to buy it for a special lady that would someday come into my life. I looked at the petite girl working in the store and asked her to put it on for size. It fit her perfectly, and I somehow knew that was the right one, so I bought it and brought it back for you."

"Allen, I'm not ready to be engaged."

"Let's just call it a friendship ring, okay?"

"Okay." Reluctantly she looked at him. "I really have to go in."

He answered, "I know. Thank you for giving me the best day of my life so far. Can I pick you up tomorrow for school?"

"I will look forward to it."

He gave her a quick kiss at the door and off he went.

As Jan started up the stairs, a terrible thought occurred to her. *This relationship is moving so fast, I know he's getting serious. Would he feel the same if he knew I'd been raped? I need to tell him the next time we're alone and have time to talk.*

She stopped at the head of the stairs, the memory of that horrible night came blasting into her mind. *He stole my virginity from me. I hate that man! How can I ever tell Allen? What man would want a used woman?* All the joy blew out of her like air escaping a balloon.

CHAPTER EIGHT

TAGS ON THEIR TOES

Part of the tour of duty during the first year of training included a visit to the morgue and observation of an autopsy. This was no doubt done with the intention to weed out the weaker students. One Friday, at the end of class, Miss Kingston randomly chose four students to go to the morgue the following Monday at seven in the morning. Jan was one of the lucky four. Since they all lived in the same dorm, it was the topic of conversation all weekend. The students knew the morgue was located in the basement of the hospital --- a frightening place regardless of the reason for being there. By the time Monday arrived, all the students pretty much had each other worked up to a fever frenzy.

They walked together from the dorm to the medical center. The gray skies and suppressive atmosphere of an impending storm reflected their own feelings. Jan made a stab at lightening their mood as she quipped, "Here we go into the dungeon." as they rode the elevator down.

Cindy gave her a disgusted look and answered, "More like a mausoleum!"

The door of the elevator slowly opened and someone behind Jan said, "Is this really mandatory because I'm about to run and hide."

Filled with fear, they giggled apprehensively as they entered the scene of every horror movie ever made. The hall was damp and dimly lit. Odd-sized pipes lined the ceiling and produced strange gurgling sounds. As the four of them walked rapidly down the hall, it seemed endless. Every dark room or sinister-looking door held a suspicious unseen monster about to jump out and attack them. As they finally turned a corner, their destination was within reach. They knocked on the door to the Autopsy Exam Room. Not receiving an answer, they slowly opened the door rather than stand outside in the scary hall.

The room was still and cold, enriching their nostrils with a variety of smells from alcohol to formaldehyde. Jan glanced around uneasily. There were three long porcelain troughs, each with a drain at one end and a hose-like apparatus at the other. There was a tube hanging down from the ceiling that looked like a scope or a tiny camera.

Cindy looked up at it and said, "Hey, I've got an idea. Why don't I lay down on the trough and one of you take my picture?"

Norma gasped, "I don't think we should. We might get in big trouble."

Jan laughed, "Norma, Cindy was joking." She turned to Cindy. "You were kidding, right?"

"Well, I was, but the more I think about it, it would make a great picture to send to some of my friends."

"I have to agree, it would be hilarious." said Jan.

They continued to look around, getting more uneasy as they waited. There were a couple of large stainless steel sinks and shelves holding different sized glass jars with human organs floating inside, reminding Jan of the anatomy lab at college. On the other side of the room was an oversized solid metal door embedded with a large round temperature gauge easily readable from across the room. A sign that read "MORGUE" and "DO NOT ENTER" in big black letters was adequate warning to stay away.

Jan thought, *I wonder if we'll be allowed to see what lays behind that door? I'm not real sure I want to.*

Cindy and the others looked as if they were ready to fly through the door. Just then, it suddenly swung open. A short, bald, mousy-looking man, dressed in a white lab coat, waltzed in wearing thick glasses that enlarged his eyes. *He could easily play the part of Frankenstein's play toy.*

"Welcome, I'm Doctor Lowry, the Chief of Pathology. I spend the greater part of my waking time in this cavernous underground dwelling." The girls stifled a giggle as he continued. "Please introduce yourselves, and then I'll show you around."

Everyone looked at Jan, so she started, "My name is Janet Winston."

"I'm Cindy Harper."

"I am Edna Franco."

"My name is Norma Shilling."

"I welcome you all to my underworld domain. Please feel free to stop me to ask questions at any time."

Dr. Lowry began explaining the equipment in the room and its various uses. He also related the reasons for the specimen jars and the sinks. He turned and walked toward the large door. "This is a refrigerated room where we store the dearly departed. They're each patiently waiting their turn for an autopsy or removal to the mortuary."

When entering, Jan felt a chill from the sudden drop in temperature. They could see seven gurneys, three empty and four others with sheets draped over the bodies. The sheets covered everything except pale gray feet with tags tied to big toes. It appeared this was a cohabitation dormitory. Jan feared that any minute one of the corpses would rise up and scare them into a run of terror!

Edna timidly asked, "Why do you tie the tags on their toes?"

She was the only student close to Mandy's height with a little more adipose tissue on her frame. She had light brown hair, hazel eyes and an attitude of superiority until she was in a group. Then she turned into a little mouse.

"That's a good question, Edna. It has a great deal to do with the shape of the large toe."

Edna let out a nervous chuckle.

"You see, fingers and all other toes are usually long and slender. Most large toes are rounder, and by tying the string at its base, it will not slide off. These people don't care where it's tied, as long as we do not misplace their identity. They're very picky about that."

They all broke out in laughter.

Dr. Lowry began to maneuver one of the occupied gurneys out of the morgue to the autopsy room. He turned to them with a pleasant smile. "Some advice before we begin. Your being here is for the purpose of educating you in the different aspects of the human body and the manifestations of disease. Dr. Lowry paused, looking at each of them individually. I will explain every step as I go through the process, and if you listen carefully, it will help take your mind off some of the more unpleasant aspects of the procedure. If the odors bother you, just breath through your mouth."

The hall door swung open, and in walked a young man, taller than Dr. Lowry and much better looking. His blue eyes and blonde curly hair reminded Jan of one of her nephews.

Dr. Lowry smiled at him. "Students, I'd like you to meet one of my assistants, Tom Fuller, who has entered at just the right time to help lift this cadaver to the exam table."

The girls stepped back as Dr. Lowry and Tom moved him into place. As they removed the sheet, the doctor told the girls to step up to the table. He paused as they moved up.

Before he could continue, Norma felt faint, and Cindy, who was standing next to her, caught her as her knees buckled. Dr. Lowry grabbed a chair, lifted her up to sit on it and put her head between her knees. He stood by her until she felt better.

As she was coming out of it, he explained further, "If any of you should feel faint, sit in one of the chairs Tom is placing around you for your convenience. Then put your head down as I have done with Miss Shilling." He then added, "You can also use one of the buckets if you should feel sick, or use the bathroom out the door and to the left."

Jan was to the side of the doctor. She was looking down at the shoulders and chest of a male adult in his early forties who had died suddenly. She felt a sense of amazement as she began to enjoy the procedure; She forced herself to ignore the offensive odor --- a mixture of stale body fluids. The doctor's explanations, seasoned with his subtle sense of humor beamed an uplifting atmosphere to the room. Janet was fascinated, seeing everything inside the body first hand. This was not anything like the formaldehyde-shriveled cadavers they had seen in anatomy lab. It was not until they took a break, prior to opening the cranium, that she realized she was the last student standing.

The autopsy lasted most of the morning. When it was finished, Dr. Lowry told them to wash up and follow him to his office across the hall. Entering the large room was like stumbling into an oasis after drifting in the barren wilderness of the desert. He had fashioned his own utopia with framed colorful photographs of various wildlife in their natural habitat. In the photos, the wildlife were standing by everything from blooming wild flowers to pine trees heavy with snow. Jan was certain he was doing his best to cover up the drab gray walls. Several bookcases held a library of reference books, tastefully adorned with artifacts and works of art. A warm pot of coffee brewed in a coffeepot in the corner. He invited them to sit down in cushiony armchairs or on the large, comfortable couch.

"Do you have any comments or questions? I will be more than happy to discuss whatever is on your mind."

Jan immediate asked, "Are there times when the only way to determine a cause of death is through an autopsy?"

"Absolutely! Good question, Janet. This happens many times. As a matter of fact, even when the doctors have diagnosed the cause by way of an autopsy, we will be able to determine other contributing factors. Pathology may be the most significant science in medicine."

"You told us during the autopsy, this man died of a severe heart attack. Wasn't he very young to have a heart attack, Doctor Lowry?" asked Cindy.

"Not when you take under consideration the extenuating circumstances. Did you notice the amount of adipose tissue in his abdomen? The amount that a person has around their heart is equal to the proportion of abdominal fat. Consequently the heart has to work overtime to force blood into the added cells, raising the blood pressure as well as other health problems. The result can be death at an early age. This man's heart literally exploded from utter exhaustion."

Norma raised her hand, "Are there very many of the nursing students that have the same adverse reaction we had during your procedure?"

He chuckled as he answered, "Frankly, this was the first time that I had three out of four respond so well to my good looks." They all laughed, and after he asked if they had any more questions, he handed them a paper signed by him to verify their attendance.

Jan held back as the others approached the door of his office. She turned to remark, "I enjoyed learning from you. Your explanations were very thorough. Thank you. Is there any possibility of observing another autopsy?"

"You are most welcome any time you're free and would like to learn more, Miss Winston, or any of the students, please feel free to do so. You must however, request permission from Miss Kingston first."

"Oh, okay thank you." She ran-walked down the hall to catch up with the others.

Later, she couldn't help but reflect, *I had such a judgmental attitude when I first saw him. He's not anything like the strange man I thought him to be. He was warm and friendly, and I would be comfortable taking him up on his offer, if Miss Kingston will approve.* She hurried to grab lunch and change so she could meet Allen for a ride to the college.

* * *

When Jan had an opportunity, she approached Miss Kingston's office. Her door was always closed which made it intimidating to knock. She tapped lightly on the door, waited a minute and started to knock louder when the door flew open and Miss Kingston looked down her nose at Jan. "Well, speak up. What do you want, Miss Winston?"

Jan's stomach churned and red blotches heated her cheeks. She stammered, "M-May I t-talk to you for a few minutes?"

"Make it one minute, I'm very busy at the moment."

Jan knew her trembling was obvious to Miss Kingston, and no effort on her part could stop it. "I need your permission to go down to see another autopsy when I have some free time."

"And may I ask why?"

"I'd like to learn more, and Dr. Lowry invited me back to watch anytime I could work it into my schedule."

"Well, since Dr. Lowry invited you, I give you my permission as long as you bring back the paper with his signature. Miss Kingston hesitated for an instant. "Miss Winston, what is it that you found so interesting?"

Caught off guard by the unexpected question, Jan took a minute to gather her thoughts. "I-I felt there was considerable value in seeing the real thing as opposed to organs in jars. I was fascinated with the procedure and observing the manifestation of disease. The heart on this man . . ."

Miss Kingston interrupted with, "And I understand that you were the only one that did not faint away. Is that true?"

With a shake of her head she answered, "Yes."

"By the way, what was it that you put in your mouth from that bedpan, Miss Winston?"

"Peanut butter mixed with chocolate syrup, Miss Kingston."

Jan looked at her and thought she might be imagining a glimmer of a smile on Miss Kingston's face. "You are showing signs of becoming an excellent student, Miss Janet Winston. Keep up the good work."

Before Jan could say another word, the door was closed. Jan walked away in a whirl of confusion, wondering if she really saw a small crack in the old lady's armor.

CHAPTER NINE
CAN'T ESCAPE FROM JOHN DOE

Jan enjoyed a few more visits with Dr. Lowry. He was always glad to see her. He shared interesting specimens and stimulated her gray matter with challenging questions.

On one of her visits he enthusiastically gushed, "Janet, you came at the right time. I have an unusual death to autopsy and I'd like you to stay."

"Tell me a little about the patient, Dr. Lowry."

"The Negro patient, twenty four years of age, entered the emergency room complaining of shortness of breath with pain radiating through his chest and abdomen. Upon examination, the doctor felt he should be admitted for further studies. They suspected a heart attack or a virus, so as a precaution he was placed in isolation while they ran several tests. His condition went from serious to critical, and he died on the fourth day."

"Oh no, how terrible!"

"Yes, it is, and they never did come up with a definitive diagnosis."

"Okay, you've piqued my curiosity."

Looking at the patient, she commented, "He's so handsome and healthy looking. It doesn't seem possible he was sick enough to die."

"You're right, Jan. That's why we do autopsies."

As the doctor opened the chest and removed the rib cage, she noticed what looked like abscesses on his lungs. The stomach revealed the same. His liver was covered with the lesions also, some the size of a man's fist.

Jan looked at Dr. Lowry and asked in a concerned voice, "Do you think this is something contagious?"

"No, I already know what it is, but I want to see if you can diagnose it before I tell you."

Jan was perplexed, but true to her nature, she loved this kind of challenge. "Right now, I don't have a clue. Had he traveled to a foreign country recently?"

"Nope."

"Was he a smoker?"

"Since the age of fourteen."

"Could it be cancer?"

"You're one smart cookie, my child! That's absolutely right; isn't it a terrible waste at such a young age? And I understand he has a wife and a small baby."

Jan cringed as she thought how many of the students smoked and many of the nurses in the hospital also.

* * *

One week later, Mrs. Jacob assigned Jan to a patient that was dying of Hodgkin's Disease. Mrs. Jacob explained, "This is a type of cancer that affects the lymph system, which you'll be studying soon. Mrs. Thompson is a fifty-three year old who has been admitted in the last stages of the disease. Mrs. Jacob looked at Jan with her expressive hazel eyes. I want you to experience the care of a terminally ill patient. I will work with you as much as my time will allow, so let's go to the room and meet her."

They entered quietly. Mrs. Thompson looked like a skeleton lying in bed, but to Jan's surprise she was very much awake and alert. She weakly raised a bony arm and said, "Please, I need a bedpan."

Mrs. Jacob and Jan answered simultaneously, "Oh, of course."

Jan reached into her bedside stand, and there was no bedpan. Mrs. Jacob looked quickly around the room and said, "Miss Winston, you'd better hurry and get one down the hall."

Jan had already started out the door, fuming that someone had not replaced a dirty bedpan with a clean one. This happened way too often.

Jan returned and placed the bedpan just in time.

What happened next was something that Jan would never forget. The patient practically filled the bedpan with a liquid stool that made her nostrils want to shrink and run for cover. The offensive odor permeated every inch of the room. Jan looked at Mrs. Jacob and she knew that her instructor was having a difficult time also. The sweet patient looked at them and said, "I'm so sorry. I really stink, don't I?"

It's okay, Mrs. Thompson; let me take the bedpan out of here, and it will help."

Fighting the urge to gag, Jan covered the pan and carried it to the Hopper Room. A Hopper was like an oversized toilet, having a receptacle to slide the bedpan into. Then a lever was pulled, rinsing it clean. Jan walked back with a clean bedpan, noticing the odor still lingered, even though Mrs. Jacob had opened a window.

Later, Jan asked Mrs. Jacob, "Why was the odor of her feces so offensive? Is it something to do with her disease?"

"It is characteristic of Hodgkin's. With the lymph system compromised, the body toxins come through the waste disposal system."

Jan gave her a complete bed bath, watching her courageously suffer with pain. She was able to give her an injection of morphine for pain, and as Mrs. Thompson relaxed she started a conversation. "Do you have any children dear?"

"No, I'm not even married yet."

"I have four wonderful children I raised as a single mom after my husband died suddenly in his mid-thirties."

"That must have been difficult for you."

"Yes, it was a struggle while they were young. But now they're all grown, and I have two sweet grandchildren. They live very far away so I don't see them often, but two of my daughters are on their way here and should arrive by this evening."

"That's wonderful. I'm sure you'll be very happy to see them."

"Yes, I just hope I can hold out until then. I feel my hours are numbered, and I keep sensing that my husband is hovering near. I have no fear of death, Miss Winston. In fact, I feel a spirit of peaceful anticipation towards my next journey. Believe it or not, I look forward to it."

"Wow, that's amazing. So many people are afraid to die."

"My faith has helped me believe in life after death and it's truly a comfort."

"You're an amazing lady." Jan said as she excused herself to get some replacement linens for her room. While she was down the hall, she stopped to dish up a small bowl of Jell-O with a few graham crackers on a tray for her patient. Upon entering her room, Jan noticed she had drifted off to sleep. She quietly put her things away. Jan heard a gasp and turned quickly to go to her bedside. She stood beside her, holding her hand. Jan asked. "Are you alright Mrs. Thompson?"

There was no response as Mrs. Thompson became very still and her eyes slowly opened, revealing a slight glaze over them. She took another short gasp of breath, and at that moment, Jan knew she had just witnessed her first death.

Jan was astounded at how peaceful she felt as she watched her drift away. She felt inclined to talk to her, even though she knew she was gone. "You've been a wonderful patient to care for, Mrs. Thompson. Your attitude toward dying has given me a good feeling about death."

Jan put her hand down and left the room. She approached an RN at the nursing station. "Mrs. Thompson in 436 has just expired. Will you page Mrs. Jacob for me?"

"Yes, I will; in the meantime, you need to procure a morgue pack from Central Supply and take it back to her room."

Mrs. Jacob came in the room right after Jan. "Miss Winston, you timed this just right. You need to go to lunch and prepare for your college classes. This time I will do the preparation of the body and send her to the morgue, but the next time a patient expires, you will be responsible to do it."

"Thank you, Mrs. Jacob and by the way, Mrs. Thompson's daughters are due to arrive this evening."

"Thanks, I'll tell the nurses."

* * *

Janet walked into the room of a "John Doe," admitted after the police found him near death in skid row. They had scrubbed him clean in the emergency room, and he seemed as contented as a newborn kitty cat after its first feeding. He was curled in the fetal position, snoring loudly with his mouth wide open. He was emaciated and looked much older than his stated age of fifty seven. His teeth were either missing or brown and jagged, his hair was a yellowish gray color and his breath would have made a hairless Chihuahua grow kinky red hair!

Jan awakened him and explained she needed to get him ready for some tests in the X-Ray department. He gave her a toothless smile and answered, "Yes Miss."

"I will give you some breakfast when you return. Please get up from the bed and step into the wheelchair so I can transfer you downstairs."

"Okay, Miss."

The orderly brought Mr. Doe back and stopped to talk with Jan. She didn't have time for chit-chat so Jan said, "I really have to get back to my patients to complete my assignment." She was helping Mr. Doe to bed when he curled over, grabbing his stomach. She thought he might get sick, so she reached for a basin. She turned back toward him, astonished; he had turned a bluish-gray color and lay limply on the bed. She turned on the call light and watched helplessly as he turned an even darker color. She couldn't find a pulse. He had stopped breathing and his eyes became glassy.

Two nurses came into the room. One of them looked at him and said, "Well he sure took a nose dive. I just saw the orderly pushing him in a wheelchair, and he looked fine!"

Jan asked, "He's dead, isn't he?"

"You got that right, Miss Winston. Here, let me show you how to close his eyes." She held both her thumbs over his eyelids. "Why don't you go page Mrs. Jacob and get a morgue pack."

Oh no, Jan thought, *I'm not going to get out of this one.*

Mrs. Jacob told her, "I'm assisting another student and will be there in five minutes. In the meantime, put him on a gurney and place him in the exam room down the hall so you can start cleaning the room."

The nurses helped to move him down the hall.

Mrs. Jacob took much longer than five minutes, and Jan finished cleaning plus completed her other patients. Her instructor apologized as they went together to the exam room. As the door closed behind them, Jan removed the sheet, brushing her hand against a bare shoulder. The patient's body temperature had dropped since moving him, triggering a flashback of a forgotten incident: Jan was five years old; her mother made her look into the casket of a neighbor and made her touch the dead woman's face. Jan had been terrified when her small hand felt the cold, hard skin. It sent a tremor of fear through her body. The memory was suddenly dissolved by Mrs. Jacob's voice.

"Miss Winston, open the pack please." They started by cleansing away body fluids that had escaped. Mrs. Jacob was standing on the opposite side of the gurney as she said, "Tell me when you're ready, and I'll turn him on his side so you can clean his back and buttocks."

"I'm ready now." Jan said.

As Mrs. Jacob pulled him over by his shoulder and hip, he let out a deep guttural moaning sound. "*OOOUUUUUUEW*!" Jan felt her knees give out, and she came down on her haunches next to the gurney. To her amazement, Mrs. Jacob had quickly let go of him and sunk to her knees as well. They were facing each other under the gurney. Jan was shaking all over when her instructor started to laugh. Jan could not hold it back, and they both laughed hysterically, gasping for breath as tears ran down their cheeks.

Once they were able to control themselves, they continued with the procedure, Mrs. Jacob explained, "The sound we heard was air left in his lungs, which escaped by turning him. That type of thing doesn't happen very often; as a matter of fact, I have heard of it and never experienced it myself until today."

Together they washed him and finished the lengthy procedure. Mrs. Jacob showed Jan how to fill out the identification tag and tie it on his big toe. Covering him with the sheet again, they called an orderly to take him to the basement. Jan was unable to attend his autopsy, but she later learned that he died of a ruptured aortic aneurysm. Jan recalled to her memory that an aneurysm is a weakening of the artery wall causing it to balloon out and can suddenly rupture, causing immediate death.

Now that Jan had experienced her first care after death, she knew she could do it again. She only hoped that from now on they would be "deadly quiet!"

CHAPTER TEN
A CROWNING GLORY

Jan ran up the stairs as fast as her legs would propel her. She turned left, ran down to Mandy's room, slid in and flopped on top of her bed. Mandy slowly turned from her desk "Have you blown a gasket? What has you so pumped up?"

Jan stretched her arms in the air. "Aren't you excited about today's news?"

"You mean the capping ceremony?"

"Of course, Mandy. We made it. We're going to be capped."

"Well, yeah, I'm happy we made it, but I must assume my enthusiasm is a bit less than yours."

"Oh, I'm sorry. Can you tell me why?"

"I just feel so bad about Edna Franco. Did you know she didn't make it?"

Jan sat straight up, running her hands through her hair. "Oh no, I didn't know. Oh my gosh, not Edna."

"Jan, why don't we go down to her room and try to cheer her up."

"That sounds like a great idea. Let's go."

As Mandy knocked on Edna's partially closed door, it slowly swung open to reveal Edna standing at her bed packing a suitcase. Edna turned towards them with tears streaming down her face. "Hi, come on in."

They rushed forward, to embrace her in a three way hug. Standing there for a minute, each searched for the right words.

Edna was the first to let go. She faced them and grabbed a handkerchief. She blew her nose and said, "I'm okay, really. I've been struggling so much with my grades. I find it difficult to relate with the patients; I honestly don't think I was cut out to be a nurse."

Jan was touched by her honesty. "Edna, you have so many valuable talents. I mean, the way you put together our skit was fantastic. I know I could never have done what you did."

"Thanks, Jan. I've already decided to go back to my local college and study dramatic arts. I know I'll feel better about myself doing something I love."

Their house mom knocked on the door. "Edna honey, your parents are here."

"Oh, tell them I'll be down in about 10 minutes."

"Edna, we just want you to know, Jan and I will miss you." Mandy said sincerely.

"Thanks, Mandy. Will you help me finish packing and assist me with my bags?"

"Absolutely."

After meeting Edna's folks, they went back to Mandy's room.

In a more somber mood Jan asked, "Mandy, who are you going to invite to our capping?"

"I don't have anyone to invite."

"What about your parents?"

Mandy lowered her eyes and spoke in a terse voice. "No, I cannot!"

Jan had never heard Mandy talk with such bitterness before. She started to ask her "why," but before the word reached her lips, Mandy quickly said, "Let's just leave it at that. I'll explain some other time."

"That's fine, Mandy. Do you have anyone else you can invite?"

"No. My only friend is sitting in my room, and that's it."

"Oh Mandy, I love you so much. You are now officially my sister and a part of my family. Does that work for you?"

"Sure, but we must have been adopted Jan, cause we sure don't look alike!"

"Really? I thought we were twins."

"You must have been drinking, my little one. You need to get a grip and study."

Jan remained puzzled by Mandy's statement about her parents, dying to ask her about it; however, she knew with time Mandy would open up to her. Jan added a small note to the invitation she wrote to her parents, asking if Mandy could be included in their family's celebration. She also mentioned that if they were bringing her a gift to bring something for Mandy to open. As an afterthought, she wrote, "She's always borrowing my Grays Anatomy."

Similar to graduation, the capping ceremony was held in the college auditorium. The remaining number of students had dwindled to twenty-four. When the evening arrived, Jan's parents came early to the dorm with Jan's older sister, Judy and her husband Rick. Jan introduced Mandy to everyone, and they hugged each other.

Jan's father interrupted. "Janet, I want you and Mandy to sit down over there." He pointed to the couch.

They sat down while her dad walked over with a beautifully wrapped large box. Jan looked at it and said, "Oh, it's so pretty, I don't want to open it!" Jan's hands trembled as she carefully took off the lovely blue bow, slowly removing the embossed wrapping paper.

Her dad remarked, "Janet, just tear it off, for Pete's sake. We don't have all day, you know."

Janet grabbed the paper and reluctantly tore it. Inside the box was a beautiful, full length, navy blue nurse's cape. As she held it up, she could see a bright red full lining. It was exquisite. Jan was speechless, amazed at such a wonderful gift. She cried with joy to think that her parents would do this for her. As she wiped away her tears, Mom said, "Jan, honey, you deserve it. Now Mandy has a gift to open from her best friend, Jan." She handed a square, heavy gift wrapped in the same exquisite paper to Mandy.

Mandy sat there holding the gift, staring.

Jan put her arm around her. "Mandy, it won't bite. Now open it!"

She took in a deep breath and slowly tore open the box. Mandy saw the label and started to cry.

"Now you can use your own Grays."

Mandy reached around and hugged Jan. She whispered in Jan's ear, "You're the best friend I've ever had. Thank you."

"You are very welcome. Now let's touch up our makeup so we can leave."

"Before you run away, are we going to meet the man you've been telling us about?" Jan's sister asked.

"He intended to be here, but his boss had an important meeting to go to, and he had to work."

"Oh, what a disappointment, Janet. When will he get off work?" Jan's dad asked.

"Not until 10:30."

"That's past my bedtime!" her mom groaned.

Jan added, "We'll make a special trip so he can meet you, I promise."

It was a chilly February night, so Jan proudly threw her warm 100% wool cape around her shoulders to wear to the ceremony. Upon their arrival, all the girls had to touch it or try it on, and Jan began to feel guilty that she was the only one with such a wonderful gift. As the baby girl in the family, she was marvelously spoiled.

The twenty four nursing students lined up to enter, twelve in each aisle. Each was handed a lighted candle in a Florence Nightingale lantern to carry as she walked down the aisle. Spaced about four feet apart, the students entered to music much like a graduation procession and climbed the side stairs onto the stage to take their seats. Jan was the first one to enter on her side, and Mandy was last to enter on the other side. Each of the instructors gave a short welcome followed by Miss Kingston. Much to the students surprise, she said some nice things about each. As their names were called, each one walked to center stage to have her nurse's caps placed on her head. It was an emotional night for all, given the work and study preceding this honor.

Monday Jan walked with Mandy, feeling like a real nurse wearing her new cap. Every RN that worked in the hospital wore a specific cap signifying their school of graduation. Jan turned to Mandy, "Of all of the different kinds of caps, I think I love ours the best."

"Not me, I feel like a flying nun." Mandy quipped.

CHAPTER ELEVEN
THE PLAYBOY HIDING BEHIND THE MASK

Jan started her rotation in the surgical department. Her instructor was waiting for her, "Welcome, Miss Winston. I'll take you to the locker room where you can change into your scrubs for the time you're here. You're not allowed to wear your cap or uniform." She said as she handed her a bundle containing scrubs.

This would become her routine for the next three months. The first week, she observed only. She learned the restrictions and interactions between the different kinds of nurses and doctors. Only RNs worked the surgical theater. At one point, she observed a laparotomy, the surgical opening of the abdomen, when an instrument went flying over her head, and some nasty words poured out of the surgeon's mouth. The surgical nurse held her tongue and turned a dark shade of purple, as her head was encircled with the steam from her ears. Jan was amazed he could get away with such a juvenile outburst. She thought *I never, ever want to assist that particular doctor.* When they were finished, she checked the board and found his name was Worthington. Filing that name in her memory bank, she went in to observe some easier procedures.

She watched a bronchoscopy, where the doctor inserts a long stainless steel tube through the larynx or voice box into the bronchus of the lungs to observe for evidence of disease. She was told she would scrub for the next one. She looked at the doctor with a question on her face, and he said, "It's okay, I don't bite, and I'll walk you through it."

Jan looked into Doctor William Marty's dark blue eyes and asked, "You mean you won't throw any instruments at me?"

He laughed heartily, and with a smile he answered, "So you've been observing Dr. Worthington?"

Jan answered with a quick nod as he remarked, "He really isn't such a bad guy, and I happen to know he is very kind to pretty student nurses."

Jan blushed and looked away.

She assisted Doctor Marty with three procedures. When they were finished he remarked, "You did very well, Miss Winston." As she turned to leave he added, "And if Dr. Worthington gives you a bad time, you tell me and I'll take him out back and rough him up a bit."

Jan laughed as she hurriedly walked out the door and ran smack into Dr. Worthington, almost landing both of them on the floor. She was so mortified, her tongue wrapped around her epiglottis! He put his hand on her shoulder and said, "Whoa there, my pretty lass. Did Dr. Marty scare you so much that you had to come out in high gear?"

Jan stammered, "N-no Sir."

He smiled and said, "Well, I'll make sure you assist me next time, and I'll treat you much better than Marty."

She didn't care for the insinuation in his voice, and she wanted to tell him she would refuse to assist him. As she turned to move away, he gave her a pat on her buttocks. Jan felt violated; even her father would never touch her there. The ugliness of rape flashed in her mind but given the status of physicians, she knew she dared not say anything. She made a fast break for it, fuming all the way down the hall.

The following week, she looked at the surgery schedule, and on Tuesday she was assigned to assist Dr. Worthington with a cholecystectomy, the removal of the gall bladder. She turned to see Miss Page coming down the hall, and Jan waved at her to indicate she needed to talk.

Miss Page was a young nurse, in her late twenties. She was about four-feet, ten-inches tall with a well-rounded figure. She wore her school's large, round cap. It nearly covered her red, curly hair. As she walked towards Jan, her curls bounced. She stopped quickly to greet Jan with a radiant smile. "Hello, Miss Winston. What do you need?"

"I need to talk to you in private."

Miss Page took Jan into an empty room, pulled two chairs together, and patted one for Jan to sit down on while she sat on the other. Jan poured out her heart. She explained in detail the incident in surgery and running into him in the hall, including his patty cake on her rear. Jan was close to tears as she continued, "Now I'm assigned to assist him tomorrow, and I refuse to work with him."

Miss Page took Jan's hand in hers as she said, "Miss Winston, as nurses, we can't always pick or choose our assignments or those we work with. Many times you will be asked to do things that may be difficult to carry out. Whether it be a patient, some family member, a nurse or a doctor that you find uncomfortable to work with, you do it anyway. You may find it easier if you take in a deep breath and say, 'Okay, I'm going to make the best of this, and I'm sure I'll learn from shouldering this assignment.' She paused to gather her thoughts. "Then when and if you become a supervisor, you will have empathy for those under your jurisdiction, and you will be able to guide them through difficult situations because you have once been there yourself. Do you understand?"

"Yes, I think so."

"Miss Winston, you cannot refuse an assignment as a student or as a graduate nurse."

"Miss Page, I don't know if I can handle it after what he did. Will you be close by tomorrow?"

"I already intended to be there tomorrow to observe. You are much stronger than you realize and I have faith in your ability to do this. Now, mind you, if there is any foolishness from the doctor, you be sure to report it to me. I will also make sure there will be another nurse in the room at all times to help keep him on his best behavior. For now, we are going to go through the surgical setup for a cholecystectomy and make sure you are well prepared."

When Miss Page opened up the cholecystectomy surgical pack, Jan was struck by the number of instruments. Miss Page explained, "The instruments are lined up exactly as Dr. Worthington wants them to be, so you need to remember to hand them to him in that order, unless he asks for something different. Remember, when the doctor puts his hand out, you must give a gentle slap with the instrument so he will feel it on his glove."

Jan had observed so many surgeries, she felt confident she could do it, her only fear was the great Doctor Worthington himself.

* * *

Tuesday came before she knew it. After changing, she walked into the scrub room to begin the lengthy cleansing preparation. Just as she started scrubbing her arms, Dr. Worthington walked in. Jan jumped as he brushed a little too close behind her to the next sink. He started his preparation. He looked her way as he said, "Well, Miss Winston, are you ready for an exciting morning spent with the best surgeon in town?"

"Of course." Jan gulped. "Are you going to be patient with me?"

He chuckled and said, "Honey, I will teach you everything you need to know and then some."

Jan made no comment to that, finished her scrub so she could enter the surgical room. The Jimmy Nurse, a non-sterile RN assigned to assist the needs of the doctor and the surgical nurse, assisted her with her gown, gloves, hat and mask.

Dr. Worthington took his position next to the patient and made an incision that started at the base of the sternum, or breast bone to the umbilicus. He then cut through the adipose tissue and moved the intestines out of the way with a couple of large retractors that another RN held in place. The doctor was a perfect gentleman, explaining each step as he went. He exposed the liver, and Jan could see an enlarged gall bladder (a small sac that stores bile to be released when fat is ingested). It looked like it was filled with multiple-sized jelly beans; the color of the sac was an abnormal sickly pale yellow.

Once it was removed the doctor explained, "While I'm already in the abdomen, I remove the appendix. I make it a practice to ask the patient prior to surgery. I haven't been turned down yet." He then demonstrated his stitching handicraft, explaining as he went, allowing her to do some stitches under his watchful eye.

When finished, Jan looked up to see Miss Page standing in the shadows on the other side of the room. Jan wondered how long she'd been there. After taking off their surgical gear, Dr. Worthington walked over to Jan. Thinking they were alone, he started to put his arm around her just as Miss Page made her presence known. He quickly dropped his arm, turning to greet her. "Well, hello Miss Page. Miss Winston caught on very rapidly and will have a great future as a surgical nurse."

She smiled as she said, "She'll have a great future in any type of nursing."

He returned the smile and remarked, "I'm going to keep her busy assisting me while she's on her surgical rotation, you can be assured of that. She adapts very well and she certainly lights up the surgical arena."

Miss Page smiled again and turned to Miss Winston saying, "Come dear, I want a full report of your experience today."

Jan followed her out of the room. Miss Page said, "You did very well. Do you feel more comfortable with him now?"

With raised eyebrows, "Yes. His explanations were thorough, and I learned a great deal."

"He's an excellent surgeon, and you can learn from him, but I do want you to experience other surgeons as well."

Janet had to make a run for it to get some lunch. She laughed as she wolfed down a plate full of raviolis covered in red sauce, after being in surgery. It didn't bother her in the least bit. She ran to change clothes and get to the bus.

* * *

Jan made it through her surgical rotation, of three months, with Dr. Worthington, and many other surgeons and staff. The nurses that worked with her asked if she would return after she graduated. Jan had enjoyed the routine of surgery, but she missed the interaction with the patients. She knew, if she did return, Dr. W. would have more on his mind than her being his surgical nurse. Oh well, she would just throw a bucket of ice-cold water on him or take Dr. Marty up on his offer!

CHAPTER TWELVE

MOTHER DEAR, YOU'RE OUT OF LINE

As soon as their nursing class convened, Miss Kingston announced, "We will not have our normal training class today, due to the birth of a severely deformed child last night. Since you have started your class in Growth and Development, I made the decision to take you to see this baby."

She paused, cleared her throat, and paced around a bit. "There are times during the development of the fetus within the uterus, the normal process will malfunction, resulting in some type of deformity. Babies can be born without arms, legs, fingers or toes. Things can go wrong with the spinal column, the brain or internal organs."

Everyone sat very still. Miss Kingston dropped her eyes to the floor and paused while she found the right words to describe what they were about to see. She finally looked up and could not hide her emotional state. With a catch in her voice she said, "In my 25 years as a nurse, I have never seen a deformity as severe as this." It appeared Miss Kingston might lose control as she continued. "It has been extremely difficult on the mother, who made the decision, against the doctor's advice, to see her baby, even though he was promptly covered with a receiving blanket and whisked away after delivery."

Miss Kingston turned to blow her nose, "What you're about to see is a full term male child, born with only the bottom part of his cranium, leaving the brain completely exposed. His eyes bulge out, his body is unusually large, weighing 16 pounds with very long arms and enlarged torso. Obviously, he was born by cesarean section."

The students glanced at each other, wondering if they really wanted to walk into this gruesome scene.

Miss Kingston paused while looking around the classroom. "Follow me to the nursery where he is in a protected area and can't be seen by others. Line up in the hall. I will then escort three of you at a time to see the baby. You may quietly move through, touch him if you desire, and take as much time as you wish. Please wait until we return to the classroom to ask questions. Let us proceed."

Jan was one of the last of the students to go in, and while waiting her turn in the hall, she watched as many of her classmates came out in tears. She tried to prepare herself to avoid being overwhelmed by her emotions. When it was time to go in, she paused in the doorway for a few seconds, slowly moving forward as the child came into full view. She walked up, not understanding why she was overcome by the desire to hold him in her arms. He just seemed so isolated and alone. She knew she wouldn't be allowed, so she took one of his hands in hers, feeling his soft skin, giving him some form of human contact. She noticed the natural inclination of a baby to curl his fingers around hers was missing. It was then she realized there was nothing she could have done to prepare herself for the feeling of emptiness akin to walking down a deserted street in the darkest night, lost in a pall of amnesia. She withdrew her hand and watched the baby moving his arms in strange circular motions. His eyes had no eyelids, which accentuated the bulging and added to his grotesque appearance. He looked huge-at least twice the size of a normal newborn. His body was pathetically monstrous. There was no evidence of pain, awareness or emotion as she stared at him; however, she was overwhelmed with her own emotions, and the tears flowed as she left the room. She knew the image of that infant would stay with her for a lifetime.

They returned to the classroom, and she was first to raise her hand and asked, "How much longer does he have to live?"

Miss Kingston drew in a quick breath, answering, "We don't think he will pull through the next 24 hours. They have purposely withheld nourishment to speed up the process." She stopped for a moment and added, "He has never cried and does not give the appearance of any amount of suffering, probably due to lack of brain activity. Without the protective cover, the brain tissue is drying out and has the appearance of being dead."

Another student asked, "Did the father see it?"

Miss Kingston simply said, "He apparently chose not to-a wise decision I might add."

Mandy asked, "Do they have any other children?"

"No. Sadly, this was their first, and based on the mother's size, they expected twins."

Another asked, "Has anyone taken a picture of him?"

"Yes, many pictures and x-rays have been taken and an autopsy will be performed, all for the purpose of further study."

Jan had to ask one more burning question. She raised her hand, "Do they know if there was anything in the parent's diet, drugs, family history or some other hazard that could have caused this?"

Miss Kingston answered, "We really don't know, but further research may shed some light on that particular question." With some hesitation she remarked, "I'm sure the parents would like some answers as well, before they attempt to have another child."

They were very subdued, each handling individual shock in their own way. Jan sensed she would not want to share this memory with anyone for a very long time.

With no more questions, Miss Kingston moved on to the announcement of their next rotation. Jan had to wait until near the last because her last name started with a "W." When "Miss Janet Winston" came out loud and clear, she went up to receive the assignment.

She sat down next to Mandy, "I'm going to the orthopedic wing, what's your assignment. Mandy whispered, "I'm going to Dr. Worthington's playground."

Jan giggled, "I'm sure you'll have more fun than I will. I'm not real excited about it. Do you know who the instructor is?"

"No, but I'll enjoy Miss Page."

"I guess I'll just wait to be surprised."

* * *

The next day Allen picked her up at noon, and asked as he drove off, "So, when am I going to meet your parents?"

"Well, they live quite a long way from here. Are you up for that?"

With his wonderful smile lighting her day, he said, "That's okay. Call them and see if we can come next Sunday. I really want to meet them. And the following Sunday we can visit my folks again."

"Make it two weeks between visits. Finals are coming up, remember?"

"Whatever you say, my little angel."

Allen took her to a small soda shop for a sandwich and a root beer float. They sat facing each other, feeling the warmth of their mutual love.

Jan became self conscious of others watching them, as she asked Allen "Why are you in such a hurry to meet my folks?"

"Honestly, I think since you have met mine, it would be nice for me to meet yours."

"Okay, Allen I understand."

Allen looked at his watch. "Hate to break this up, but it's time to go to class."

In the car, Allen reached over, pulling Jan to him. "We have a couple of minutes left" he said as he kissed her tenderly. Releasing his arm around her waist momentarily, he whispered, "You sure know how to put me into a tailspin!" Then pulled her in again for another longer kiss before driving away.

He dropped her off close to her class, exclaiming, "Our time together is never enough!" and he went around to park. Jan was lost in thoughts of Allen's kisses as she walked to class. She entered the classroom, smiling from ear to ear.

Mandy leaned over when Jan sat down and said, "What did you and Allen do on your lunch hour?"

"Had lunch, and I'll tell you the rest later."

Allen had to work, so she rode back on the bus and told Mandy what Allen wanted to do next Sunday.

When they arrived at the dorm, Jan called home. "Hi Daddy, you're just the one I wanted to talk to."

"Well that's nice. You know I'm always eager to talk to my sweet daughter."

"Is everything okay with you and mom?"

"Sure. She's just giving me the evil eye 'cause I got to the phone first."

"Sounds normal. Do you and mom have any plans for Sunday?"

"Mother, do we have any plans on Sunday, other than going to church?"

Jan could hear a muffled answer. "Mom says all's clear, but she is getting nosy and wants to know why."

"My boyfriend, Allen, wants to meet you, he suggested we drive up on Sunday."

"Sounds exciting. We'll have an early dinner for you. Sound good?"

"Absolutely! We will see you Sunday, okay?"

"Do you know how to get here?

"You're real funny, Daddy!"

"Just wanted to make sure. It's been awhile."

"Gotta go. Love you and we'll see you Sunday."

"Can hardly wait."

Now Jan was really excited, she had to wait to call Allen after work. When she told him, he was ecstatic. It was a shame they had to wait until Sunday, and this was only Wednesday. Jan found it difficult concentrating on her studies, Mandy always had a calming influence on her to help settle her down. She was so grateful for their friendship.

* * *

Allen picked up Jan early Sunday and they started their journey to her folks. "Tell me a little about your folks, so I know what to expect."

"Wait a minute. That's not fair. You told me zip about your parents before I met them!"

"You got me there, but this is different."

"And what is the difference, Mr. Allen?"

"Well, Miss Janet, I knew my mother would be captivated by your beauty and charm, and I didn't need to program you ahead of time."

"Well, you have charm and you're very handsome. Oh, okay, I'll tell you about my parents. They've been married close to 40 years, and they have three children. My brother is the oldest, then my sister Judy and me. Mom has always been a housewife and mother. My dad is a very successful businessman. He owns a retail store in town that sells office equipment, furniture and stationary. He also repairs typewriters and adding machines.

"I think it's neat you have a brother and sister. I missed out on that being the only child."

"Yeah, it's nice, but they're both a lot older than me. By the time I graduated from grammar school, they were both gone. My folks live in a very old home that has been remodeled from the foundation up. They furnished it in mostly antiques. Do you like antiques?"

"I don't know much about them, to tell you the truth, but I have an aunt that has a lot of them."

"Wait till you see my folks. They have some really neat ones, and there's a story behind every one."

"I bet your dad is very protective of his little girl."

"Oh, I guess so. I do know he's very strong."

"Now you're making me shake in my boots."

When they finally arrived and introductions were over, her parents had a million questions for both of them, and then her dad concentrated on Allen. Jan was sure Allen must have felt like he was on the witness stand at a hot trial, but he answered with honesty and his genuine personality. He even opened up about his own dad. Jan could tell her father was really warming up to him. She felt good all over.

While the men were talking, her mom suggested she and Jan go in the kitchen to check their meal. Her mom closed the door, and they sat at the small breakfast table. "Jan, honey, I want to tell you how impressed I am with Allen. He's extremely good-looking, and I can tell there is a real connection between the two of you."

"Yes, mom, there certainly is, and I bet it shows!"

"Jan, I want you to be perfectly honest with me. Have you had sex with him?"

"Mom, you know me better than that. Absolutely not! Not even close. All we've done is kiss!"

"Have you been alone with him in his room?"

"Mother, no! Don't you trust me?"

"Yes, but I had to hear it from the horse's mouth. I am well aware of the challenges you face with a long term relationship when there is such electricity between you. It reminds me of how your dad and I felt before we were married."

"Mother, are you saying that you did?"

"Did what?"

"Have sex?"

"Of course not!"

"Well then I don't think this conversation was necessary."

Her mother reached over to hug her with misty eyes and said, "I suppose not, and I'm sorry. Forgive me?"

"Oh mom, of course, but don't you ever ask me again."

"I promise, now tell me more about Allen."

"Mom, he treats me like I'm very special, and he has a terrific sense of humor. Let's go back to the living room so you can get to know him for yourself." Jan rose from the table.

"Okay, let me just check the roast and I'll be right in."

As Jan walked out she thought, *"I'm well aware that my mother can be very outspoken, but I didn't expect her to drop the 'S' bomb."*

The rest of their time together was great; they all had a lot of laughs when Jan filled them in on some of her nursing escapades. The folks took them out for a short ride, showing Allen the town and her dad's business. Jan apologized for having to leave early, but studies came first.

On the way home, Allen said, "I can't get over how nice your parents are, and your father is really a great person, a lot like my dad before the accident. But I still want to see my folks in two weeks. Is that okay?"

"I have to be honest. I would much rather just see your mom."

"I agree. Maybe if we're lucky she'll be the only one there."

Jan floated up to her room as she always did after spending a day with Allen. She tried to clear her mind so she would be able to concentrate on her studies.

Mandy had left a note to come down to her room when Jan came in, so she picked up her books and double stepped down the hall.

"Hey, you look happy." said Mandy.

"Mandy, I just spent the day with Allen and my parents. What did you expect?"

"I expect you to tell me every detail of your day."

"Well, let's see. We drove, we talked, we visited, we ate and we drove again."

"Oh, how did you possibly do all of that in just one day?"

"My mom asked me if we were having sex."

"NO, she didn't!"

"It's okay. I set her straight. Mandy, I really think my folks liked him. The only negative thing my mom mentioned was his gum chewing. It bothers me too, but I'm trying to get used to it."

"Well, chewing gum is better than picking his nose!"

Jan giggled, "Yes, I suppose so, but I know my dad liked him. He talked to him for quite awhile. Then, when we left, my dad leaned into Allen and whispered something in his ear."

"Wonder what that was about."

Jan was lost in a blank stare when Mandy cleared her throat. "Jan, come back to Earth. We need to study."

"Okay, but now I have to endure another visit with his folks in two weeks, why would he want to go back so soon?"

"Jan, study!"

"Okay. Pharmacology, right? Let's see if we can come up with a concoction to make me excited about working on orthopedics, okay?"

"Let's do it."

CHAPTER THIRTEEN
MICHAEL

Miss Janet Winston stepped off the elevator on the fifth floor to orthopedics. At the nurse's station, she saw Miss Kingston standing behind the desk laughing with one of the nurses. Jan, now a junior, had never seen Miss Kingston laugh. She often thought Miss K was born with a permanent frown painted on her face. *So she does have a side she hides from her students.*

As a junior, Jan wore a white stripe on her sleeve and a class pin that was attached to the left-hand corner of her cap. Having accomplished this milestone, she also knew more was expected of her. As she stood waiting for Miss Kingston to acknowledge her, she was pleased to see a number of patients in the halls. Some were in wheelchairs, a few on crutches and many using walkers. Some were a bit younger than on the other floors; she guessed sports injuries played a role.

She turned back to the nurse's station just as Miss Kingston cleared her throat. "Miss Winston, welcome to orthopedics. I hope you will enjoy it as much as I do."

Miss Kingston turned to introduce Jan to the nurses, "I'd like you to meet Miss Winston who will be here for the next 2 months. Miss Winston, meet Mrs. Beckstrom and Miss Kidman. They will help you when I'm not available."

"I'm happy to meet you." Jan said.

"Now I will take you on a tour." Miss Kingston moved around easily while she showed Jan the various places devoted to care of the patients. They entered a large area dedicated to physical and hydrotherapy.

Jan turned to Miss Kingston, "This is quite impressive. Will I be able to work in here?" "Absolutely, Miss Winston and I'm sure you will enjoy it."

Something new to Jan was the use of a Stryker frame --- an apparatus used for patients with fractured neck vertebrae and spinal cord injury. Jan was fascinated by the structure --- and petrified to think she'd ever use it.

Miss Kinston explained, "A Stryker frame holds the patient rigid and permits turning to various angles without individual motion of body parts. The device supports two rectangular pieces of lightweight but strong material. One side is on the anterior, or front side of the patient and the other on the posterior, or back side. The patient is held firmly between the canvases like being in a sandwich. The device may then be rotated to position the patient on his or her back or stomach. This permits the nurses to turn the patient without his or her assistance, keeping the spine rigid. After a turn is completed, the uppermost portion of the frame can be moved away from the patient. The frame itself sits inside a very large circular, sturdy structure which supports its movement.

Miss Kingston looked at Jan and sensed her fear. "Miss Winston, before you are assigned to care for a patient in this frame, you will have experienced it yourself, and you will be given all of the practice you need to handle it properly. Come, let's move to the next room and meet a patient who is currently in one."

Together they stepped out in the hall and walked into the next room. A young man was on his back with an apparatus fastened to the frame that was holding a book for him to read. As they entered, he said to Miss Kingston, "Well, hello gorgeous. It's about time you came to see me, it looks like you brought a surprise package." He grinned at Jan.

Miss Kingston smiled, "Michael, this is Miss Winston, one of my student nurses, and if you don't behave yourself, I'll teach her how to drop you to the floor!"

"Well, you're being feisty today. Did you get up on the wrong side of the bed, Miss K?"

Without missing a beat, Miss Kingston walked over to the frame and sternly asked, "How long have you been on your back?"

A nurse walked in answering, "Just over an hour. He's well done. We need to turn him."

Miss Kingston stepped forward saying, "Let's do it. He's about ready for an attitude adjustment."

Janet watched while the two nurses flipped him over like a perfectly golden brown pancake. It looked so easy, she thought and couldn't help laughing out loud when Miss Kingston got down on her knees and looked up at Michael as she quipped, "How's the weather up there?"

Michael chuckled and said, "Watch out. I might drop my teeth on you!"

As Miss Kingston lifted herself off the floor, she patted him on his shoulder, "I'll be back later to give you a bad time."

Miss K and Jan walked out the door, Mike retorted, "Don't you always?"

Jan was flabbergasted. All this time, Jan thought Miss Kingston didn't have a funny bone in her entire body. She was amazed at what she had heard and seen. Jan was a little afraid to ask, but she decided to anyway. "Miss Kingston, have you worked a lot on orthopedics?"

Miss Kingston actually smiled at Jan as she answered, "My dear, most of my career has been spent on this floor. When I went back to earn my teaching degree to become an instructor in the nursing program, my heart remained on the fifth floor. I will be monitoring your rotation as well as the other students in orthopedics probably until I retire. Now come. I have more to show you."

One of the first patients was laying in bed with a traction device to take pressure off her spine. Miss Kingston said, "Darlene, this is Miss Winston. She will be caring for you tomorrow."

As they walked out, Jan asked, "Why are we allowed to call a patient by their first name? Isn't that against the rules?"

"Miss Winston, orthopedics is like a whole different world. When a patient is admitted here, they are asked how they want to be addressed-first or last name. It's as simple as that."

"Why don't we do that in the rest of the hospital?"

"Frankly, I don't know. This was only established here about a year ago. Maybe they're waiting to see if it works here before allowing it elsewhere."

Jan was happy to see Darlene in the morning; she took care of four other patients as well. One of her patients was in a total leg cast that had to be elevated at all times with an overhead traction. He required a complete bed bath. She reflected on the difference in orthopedic patients. The patients were very knowledgeable about their own devices and care. It was a fun floor to work on and a refreshing atmosphere.

After two weeks on the floor, Miss Kingston transferred her to the Physical Therapy Unit. Miss K. said, "Bring a bathing suit to go in the hydrotherapy pool. You'll be assisting with patients in the pool."

The therapist made sure she experienced all the treatments from hot waxing to balancing with resistance. She learned so much, it gave her a new perspective of therapy. She soon was able to do many of the treatments herself.

She was pleased to see Michael brought in and carefully lowered into the warm water. Giving him a high sign, she went over to him. "Hi Michael, how are you doing?"

"Hey, hi there, Miss Winston. I've been meaning to thank you for stopping by once in a while and lighting up my dreary room."

"You know I enjoy visiting with you. It won't be long, and I'll be able to swing you into a cartwheel myself."

"Do you think Miss K. will let you take care of me?"

"I'm counting on it."

Jan observed for awhile and then was allowed to help with his exercises. She stretched and massaged his atrophied muscles.

"Do you think I'll ever be able to walk again, Miss Winston?"

"I wish I had a magic wand and could tell you to walk out of here today, but only the doctors can answer that, Mike."

"I know, but if I can't, I want you to start perfecting that magic wand."

"For you, I will do just that."

"Would you like to hear how I got myself into this predicament?"

"If you want to tell me, of course I would."

"A few months ago, in celebration of my twenty-first birthday, my buddies and I hiked to a remote area of the Sierra Nevada mountains. We set up camp next to an isolated body of water called Asa Lake. It's fed by an artesian well, bubbling pure fresh water out of granite rocks. We rigged a rope swing to propel us over the rocks and into the deeper water. We were having a great time, drinking and swinging into the water.

Michael paused, choked up a bit. "I don't remember the rest of this. The guys told me afterward. I guess I took a running jump for the rope. My hands slipped off, and I crash landed in the rocks, breaking my neck." He looked at Jan. "That was a pretty stupid thing to do, wasn't it?"

"Michael, we all do stupid things sometimes. The only thing is, some end up with devastating results. What if you'd been drinking and driving? You could have killed a couple of your buddies and still have ended up like you are now. You would feel a lot worse, wouldn't you?"

"Yeah, you're right. Anyway, they say I was knocked out, and they were afraid I would drown! Four guys struggled to carry me on the slippery rocks. They made a stretcher from a sleeping bag and carried me several miles to our vehicle. One of the guys rolled up some clothing to brace each side of my neck."

"Do you realize doing that probably saved your life, Mike?"

"No wow, I guess I should thank them. Anyway, they drove me to the hospital, knowing any minute I could die. The doctor's rushed me into surgery. These tongs were screwed into the top of my skull to hold me in my fancy new swing. They say I will never walk again. I guess I'm lucky I can breathe and talk on my own!"

Jan helped transfer Michael back to his room. The nurses left, and before Jan went back to the nurse's station she commented to him, "Michael, you have such a great attitude."

"I can thank Miss K. for it. I was really nasty when I first got here. I was mad at God and the world. She verbally knocked me to my senses, telling me how my attitude was preventing a good recovery. She read me the riot act without pulling any punches. It turned me around and here I am."

"Well, I'm glad she did it, 'cause I really like you just the way you are.'

"Great! Now, will you marry me?"

"Sure, but I'll have to talk it over with my boyfriend first."

"Spoilsport!"

Jan laughed on her way to the nursing station. She sat down in a chair, and Miss Kingston walked in saying, "Miss Winston, follow me." Miss K. stopped next to Michael's room, where there was an empty Stryker frame. "We're going to let you experience the frame for awhile"

Jan wanted to say "no" but that wasn't an option. "Yes, of course," Jan answered.

Miss Kingston positioned Jan on the canvas, "Now hold your head rigid as though you were in the tongs." Once Jan was settled in, the nurses placed the other part on top of her and she momentarily felt like she might smother. Jan closed her eyes, feeling them turn her over like on a Ferris wheel. She experienced momentary disorientation, and was not sure if she was up or down. Jan slowly opened her eyes, and all she saw was the floor. They didn't remove the top part --- without it she could jump right off. Miss Kingston said, "Okay, we'll see you in a little bit."

Jan felt a sense of helplessness being dependent on others to rescue her. The minutes ticked away as she worked to suppress the temptation to scream for help. It seemed an eternity. Jan calmed her nerves by thinking about Allen. She loved his personality and giggled as she thought about his sense of humor. He was such fun to be with. The only thing driving her nuts was his addiction to gum. He was always chewing it.

Jan jumped at the sound of Miss Kingston's voice, "Are you ready to be released from your captivity?"

"I can't wait to get out of this thing!"

Miss Kingston chuckled and went to work removing the apparatus.

Jan was now confident with the Stryker frame and Miss Kingston had her give an in-service presentation to the other students.

Near the end of her rotation in orthopedics, Jan was assigned to Mr. Dewey, a double amputee. Jan was familiar with Mr. Dewey, having cared for him before, and never had any problem. He had developed an infection in one of his stumps which would require a dressing change. "It's time for my Demerol shot, and I need it now!" Mr. Dewey said in a demanding tone.

Jan had not even said, "Good morning," so she smiled nicely and said, "Mr. Dewey, I will have to check your chart, and if it's time, I will bring it back for you."

He raised his voice a notch and said, "I know it's time. Now go get it!"

Jan walked out thinking *He's sure on a roll this morning!*

She proceeded to the nurse's station, checked the current orders and walked to the med cabinet. One of the RNs held out a syringe for her and said, "I just mixed it for him. Here you can give it."

The students had been giving injections for quite some time, and she was familiar with the technique of mixing drugs. However Jan had been taught never to administer any medication that someone else had mixed. She looked at the RN and said, "I'm not allowed to give an injection another nurse has prepared."

The RN just stared at her and with a syrupy, disgusted voice answered, "You can give this. It's only sterile normal saline!"

Miss Winston stared back and asked, "Why are you giving him saline?"

The RN suddenly changed her disgusted look while staring over Jan's head.

Then she heard Miss Kingston's voice, "Miss Winston, what seems to be the problem?" Turning around to face her instructor, Jan answered, "I think you need to ask Nurse Perry about it."

Miss Kingston shifted her eyes to the nurse. "Will you explain the situation here?"

"All I did was offer her a syringe I had filled with sterile saline to give to her patient."

"And what did my student do?"

"She refused."

Miss Kingston's eyebrows rose into a tight arch while staring at the RN over Jan's head. She walked over to the nurse, took the syringe from the nurse's hand, squeezing the liquid into the sink. She turned back to Jan and said, "Now why don't you start from scratch, Miss Winston, just as you've been taught."

Jan turned back to the med cabinet to sign out a Demerol tablet. She counted just one, placing it in the open syringe. She then inserted the plunger and filled it with sterile normal saline to melt the tablet. She rocked the syringe back and forth to make certain the tablet had been absorbed by the saline.

Nurse Perry spoke up in a meek voice to Miss Kingston, "The doctor was just here and gave me a verbal order to start weaning him from his Demerol with every other injection being plain saline."

The RN knew she was in more hot water as Miss Kingston said, "And have you written the order in the chart?"

With her eyes taking in a wide view of the floor, the nurse could barely be heard saying, "No, not yet."

"Then until the order is written, my student will give him the Demerol. And by the way, don't ever give another nurse or one of my students a syringe you have filled and tell them to give it. And since you were one of my students a few years back, I'm very much aware that you know better!"

Realizing that Miss Kingston was really hot under the collar, Jan made a quick exit to give his injection. The patient mellowed out in short order and continued to be pleasant for the rest of the morning. Four hours later, he was asking for another "fix," and now that the order had been written, Jan gave him his placebo.

Jan was there just long enough to see that, because he was unaware of the change, he mellowed out just as though he had received the real thing. This surprised her to see that a little bit of nothing could have the same effect as a little bit of something.

A couple of days later she was taking care of a very pleasant thirty-year-old gentleman who had been admitted for observation after a small tractor had rolled over him, fracturing his leg, with the added possibility of internal injuries. She had already given him his morning care when he told Jan he was kind of tired and thought he would take a nap.

She was cleaning up around his unit when she heard him moan. Jan looked up and saw him lose consciousness and turn cyanotic. She ran to his bedside, pushed the call light and felt for a pulse. There was none. She then did the only thing that came to her mind. She leaped onto his bed, straddled him, made a fist and hit him on the chest about where his heart was. He jerked, opened his eyes and took in a startled breath. Jan jumped off just as a nurse and doctor appeared.

She felt some embarrassment regarding her actions as she explained exactly what had happened. The doctor complimented her and said she had done just what he would have done. She was so grateful she had not hesitated and had reacted to a strong gut feeling.

Jan Winston left the orthopedic ward grateful for the experience. She had not only enjoyed getting to know Miss Kingston, but she had learned many things she would take with her for the rest of her nursing career.

She walked out feeling at least an inch taller-well maybe she just wanted to be. She had no idea where her next rotation would take her, but in her wildest imagination Jan could not have predicted the emotional roller coaster ride to come.

CHAPTER FOURTEEN

THE PIERCING SCREAMS

Watkins Medical Center was one of the largest hospitals in the United States. There were parts of it Jan had never entered. The hospital was six stories high with eight elevator shafts-four in the middle for visitors and two at each end of the ward halls for transporting patients. Large wings behind the hospital were used for iron lung patients, contagious diseases, geriatrics, psychiatric, etc. At the very end of this massive structure was a large building separate from all of the rest. Gray with black trim, similar to the architecture of the nurse's dormitory, two stories with many windows upstairs. It was surrounded by large bushes and trees covering parts of the view.

When Jan was on the fifth floor, she could see the building across the courtyard and wondered if she would ever step inside. It seemed a mysterious shield surrounded the building giving the appearance of being impenetrable. She and two other students would report to this strange place on Monday.

Sunday, she and Allen spent a couple of hours together between studying for exams and his job at a gas station. After he picked her up, she shared her apprehension: "Allen, I'm very concerned about my next rotation."

"And why is that, Jan?"

"There isn't much to tell. All I know is I am going there tomorrow morning with two other students, and I know where the building is, but I don't know what's inside."

"Where's the building?"

"In back of the main hospital grounds, but not connected to it, kind of like the dorm."

"Can we get to it, Jan?"

"I suppose so, but I've never tried."

"Well, let's do it."

He drove out the main drive and circled around the hospital to see if they could find a back way. As they meandered their way around the streets behind the hospital, they found a nice clean neighborhood of older, well-kept, small homes. Allen spoke first.

"Do you find it rather odd? Every house is painted exactly alike-the same colors as the large building and your dorm."

"It certainly is strange. I wonder why."

Allen found a parking area at the back of the building; however, there was a very high wrought iron fence between them and the building. Allen and Jan could see picnic tables and benches sitting on a well- manicured green lawn between the fence and the building. "You know what, Jan? I think the fence only surrounds the large backyard."

Jan turned to Allen and said, "What do we do now?"

Looking at her with a raised eye brows, he answered in a high pitched witch's voice, "Just follow me, my little pretty!"

She put her hand in his, and off they went down a well worn path overgrown with bushes and stately trees as they sang, "Lions and tigers and bears, oh my." They rounded a corner as the side of the structure came into view, overwhelming them with its austere presence. Not wanting to go past the front, they decided to double back on the path and walk around to the other side of the edifice. While walking, they were impressed with the enormous length of the structure. When they reached the other side, they stared up at the building, Jan thought she heard children whimpering.

She turned to Allen. "Did you hear that?"

"Yes. What do you suppose it means?"

Jan looked at the windows upstairs and saw that two of them were slightly open. She started to answer when they were astounded by a child's piercing scream!

Allen put his arms around Jan as she flew into his embrace. "What in the world are you getting yourself into, Pumpkin?" he asked.

Jan could hardly find her voice, "I guess I'll find out tomorrow." He kept his arm around her as they walked back to the car. Neither spoke as they drove back to the dorm, but before Jan got out of the car, Allen said, "Jan, you be careful tomorrow, and I'll pick you up at lunchtime. I have a feeling you'll have a lot to tell me."

Jan leaned over and gave him a quick kiss, "Okay, I can hardly wait to see you at noon."

She walked into the dorm with a feeling of doom. On the second floor, Cindy came running down the hall, "Did you know that we're going together to that weird building tomorrow?"

Jan was taken aback at Cindy's obvious excitement and unusual friendliness and thought it would be wise to tell her what she had just experienced. "I think you had better come into my room so I can share something with you."

Cindy jumped in the middle of Jan's bed as Jan turned her desk chair to face her.

Jan told her the whole story of what she and Allen had found, then added the last bit of horror.

Cindy looked startled and asked, "What do you think it was? Some kind of torture chamber or something?"

"I really don't know, Cindy, one thing it brought to mind is that it may be a home for psychotic children. We just finished our semester in psychology, and Mr. Herbert talked about children with different kinds of psychoses that cannot be controlled in a normal home environment, remember?"

"Yes, I do, but please tell me there is a way we can get out of this!" Cindy exclaimed.

Jan was momentarily distracted as she looked at Cindy with her blonde, natural wavy hair surrounding a perfect heart-shaped face with big, round, gorgeous green eyes and naturally long eyelashes. Cindy was a little taller but easily the same dress size. Jan thought *She is really pretty*! Jan was pleased with Cindy's friendliness toward her. Mandy had been right about her coming around. Jan asked Cindy, "Do you know who our instructor will be?"

Cindy turned her head to the side, with a silly grin she ventured a guess. "What if it's Mrs. Stewart?"

Jan stood up from her chair groaning, throwing herself on the bed next to Cindy. "Oh no, do you think?" Jan remembered her only too well in the lab and classroom. "Do I ever!"

Mrs. Stewart was obsessive compulsive, always picking at every little thing. She drove everybody crazy, even the other instructors. Jan would prefer Miss Kingston any day. "Cindy, please say it can't be true."

Cindy was holding her sides laughing at Jan when Mandy walked into the room. "What's going on in here?"

So once again, Jan reiterated all that had transpired with Allen and then Cindy. Mandy started to giggle, "It is Mrs. Stewart!" She could hardly stop laughing as she continued, "I overheard her talking to Miss Kingston about it. Apparently this is a new assignment for her, and she doesn't like it one little bit."

"We are going to a loony bin with a loony!" Jan covered her face and couldn't stop laughing.

The three girls laughed their way, arm in arm, to the cafeteria for dinner. After they were seated, others came to their table and everyone joined in more laughter. When the conversation lagged, one of the girls looked at Jan and asked, "Hey, Jan, when are you and that gorgeous man going to tie the knot?"

Jan was startled by the change of subject. As she caught her breath, she squeezed out, "He hasn't even asked me yet, and besides, I won't get married until after I graduate."

Moans and groans were heard around the table. Another said, "You're not going to make him wait for 'you know what' are you?"

Before Jan could answer, Cindy popped up and said, "There is no way she could possibly wait with a man like him. He is some kind of sexy!" Then she added, "Hey, Jan, if you are holding out, just send him to my room."

That ruffled Jan's feathers a bit, and she responded, "Cindy, please understand that Allen and I decided a long time age to wait until we're married. I'm not saying that's always easy, but it's what we both want. Okay?"

Quiet filled the room, subduing the girls' laughter. To ease the sudden tension, she added, "But you will all be invited to the wedding after we graduate-if he asks me."

They responded with clapping and whistling as they got up to return to the dorm.

Cindy purposely followed Jan into her room and closed the door behind her. Jan turned to Cindy, and she could tell Cindy was in a somber mood. Cindy looked at Jan and asked, "How do you do it?"

"Do what?"

"Keep from having sex with a man?"

Sensing Cindy's sincerity, Jan sat down on the bed with her and answered, "I don't know. I was taught high moral standards from the time I was a little girl. I guess I just made up my mind a long time ago that I would abide by those morals."

"But doesn't he ever try?"

"No, he never has. We also make sure that we are not put into a compromising position. As an example, I have never been to the place where he lives alone in a rented room and bath. We always meet in public places."

Cindy giggled a little and asked, "What about his car? You're alone there."

"In a car! Cindy, you have to be kidding!" Then she paused, "Cindy, have you seen the size of his car?" Jan doubled over with laughter.

"Could we have a long talk together soon, Jan, when we're not so busy studying."

Jan hugged her, "Sure, any time."

As Cindy left the room Jan giggled, "Can't wait for our big adventure into never-never land."

CHAPTER FIFTEEN
SHE'S A NURSE?

Following breakfast, a subdued Janet, Cindy and Kimberly walked the distance to the mysterious building. There was a familiar feeling in the air of a warm summer day. As they approached, they saw Mrs. Stewart standing at the large ornate front door that looked like an entrance to a mystical castle. Cindy grabbed Jan's hand and gave it a knowing tug. Mrs. Stewart was older than Miss Kingston, almost as tall and wore her dyed black hair in a bun. They could easily have been sisters, but no one dared to ask.

They went up the few stairs to Mrs. Stewart. Without any acknowledgment of their arrival, Mrs. Stewart handed each of them a key with a number on it and said, "You will need a key to get through the front door as you serve your rotation here. The keys must be accounted for and returned to me on your last day. Do you understand?"

They answered in unison, "Yes."

"Now come inside, and don't forget to wipe your feet on the mat."

They entered a lobby area that was decorated similar to their dorm, as Mrs. Stewart gestured for them to sit on one of the couches.

"'This is a home for children placed for custodial care. You will be exposed to every degree of mental retardation, psychoses, and debilitating deformities. These children come from all over the state to be housed here. Most of them have been placed soon after birth. Once their problems are recognized by a physician, they recommend removal from the home. Parents are then free of their obligation and can spend time with normal members of their family. No one should be burdened with an abnormal child."

Mrs. Stewart looked at each one of them without a hint of a smile. "You will be required to feed, clean up their messes and pick up after them. These children are unable to have a one-on-one relationship. They are incapable of giving or receiving love. Your job will be to keep them clean. Now I will take you around to meet the staff, and for today you will observe only. Tomorrow you will receive an assignment. Any questions?"

Jan shivered and rubbed her arms. These were little children for heaven's sake! Certainly they had feelings and needed nurturing. She knew it was best to remain quiet, avoiding foot-in-mouth disease around Mrs. Stewart. Cindy and Kimberly just stared. Jan couldn't help but wonder if they had the same feelings.

Jan looked forward to working with Kim. She was the only student shorter than Jan. She had a perfect figure, expressive brown eyes and the most beautiful thick, silky black hair with a hint of red highlights. Her features were perfect, and she sparkled with good humor. Jan enjoyed being around her.

They trailed down a hall behind Mrs. Stewart and entered a large area where children were being fed. They stopped for a minute to observe and Jan couldn't help but notice the children's hands were being held down by the worker's free hand. Some were noticeably agitated, trying to wrestle their hands free. This really bothered Jan.

Mrs. Stewart then introduced them to Miss Ripley, the supervising RN who was in charge of the entire building. Miss Ripley seemed reluctant to greet them when introduced, quickly raising her head, with a sober face, curtly said hello and put her head back down to her work. Miss Ripley was considerably obese; her face was covered with acne, and her head was topped off with a crown of unruly bleached blonde hair.

They started down the hall, and noticed large wards on each side, many of them filled with over-sized cribs. Jan stopped at one room, and stared at an older child, resting on her side with an enormous sized head. She couldn't help being drawn to her. Mrs. Stewart spoke in a harsh tone. "Miss Winston, what do you think you're doing?"

Jan quickly turned answering, "May I go in and talk to her?"

"She won't be able to talk. It's a waste of valuable time!"

"Can I just get a closer look?"

"Go ahead, if you're so curious."

Jan went up to her crib and reached her own hand between the bars to touch her outstretched hand.

Mrs. Stewart talked with a loud, shrill voice. "You must remember to wash your hands before and after even the slightest touch of these children. You never know where their filthy little hands have been. Do you understand? Remember cleanliness is next to Godliness!"

Cindy rolled her eyes behind Mrs. Stewart's back.

Jan hurried to wash her hands then approached the little girl. "You are very pretty."

To Jan's surprise, she answered in a soft voice. "Are you my nurse?" The pupils of her eyes moved rapidly from side to side. Jan could see she was able to move her upper extremities, but her legs were extremely small and deformed.

"No, not today, honey. Can you tell me your name?"

"I'm Sandra, what's yours?"

"Oh, what a nice name. I'm Jan."

Mrs. Stewart loudly cleared her throat. "We only use our proper titles and our last names, Miss Winston!"

Jan winced as she winked at Sandra, saying, "That's right, I am Miss Winston. Can you tell me how old you are, honey?"

"I'm eight."

"Wow," Jan said. "Have you been here a very long time?"

"Enough chit chat," Mrs. Stewart interrupted. "We need to move on!"

Jan quickly told Sandra, "I'll be back to visit you real soon." *Without Mrs. Stewart, I hope,* she thought.

Before leaving the room, Jan could see many other children and babies with varying degrees of enlarged heads.

Mrs. Stewart hurriedly took them down the hall to a stairway where they climbed to the second floor. She introduced them to another RN. "This is Miss Potter."

Miss Potter was very attractive, with natural blonde hair to her shoulders and lovely blue eyes. She smiled and said, "Welcome to Watkins Home. We will try to make your stay as enjoyable as possible."

A group of children came up the stairs with a couple of caretakers herding them along.

As soon as Mrs. Stewart saw the children, she turned to us and said, "I must leave now. Remember that today you are just to observe. You are free to go anywhere as long as you do nothing more than observe the children. I will meet you here in the morning to get you started."

As she turned to go down the stairs, she stopped one of the caretakers and asked in an authoritative voice, "Did you wash their hands and faces before you brought them upstairs?"

The lady said, "Yes, of course."

Mrs. Stewart took a child by the hand and in a rebuking voice said to the caretaker, "Well, either you were careless with this one or you didn't do him at all. Now go and wash him immediately!" She thrust the child away and stomped down the stairs.

Jan, Kim and Cindy watched in complete silence, mortified and embarrassed at their instructor's behavior. Cindy muttered under her breath, "Can we tell the children that we don't know her?" They all giggled to release the tension.

Jan went down to Miss Potter and asked, "Do you have time to answer a couple of questions?" "Of course. I'd be happy to."

"These children seem more active than downstairs. What is the major difference?"

"The children must be ambulatory to live up here. We have no elevator. Most of these children suffer from some form of mental retardation or psychiatric disorder. Those that are downstairs may have similar diagnoses coupled with deformities that keep them from using stairs."

She smiled, "You girls can go into any of the rooms, observe or interact with the kids. Feel free to come to me if you have any questions."

"Thank you, we will probably have a million of them." *We certainly can't ask our instructor.*

The girls wandered down the hall, watching the interaction between the caretakers and the children. While they stopped outside of one of the rooms, they were suddenly startled by that same high-pitched scream coming from down the hall.

Miss Potter noticed their reaction and walked over to them saying, "It's alright, girls. Little Katrina is not being tortured. She is deeply disturbed and unable to communicate other than what you just heard. Would you like to meet her?"

"Oh yes," Katrina was five years old, but only about the size of an average three year old. She was a beautiful child with almost translucent, pale white skin, light red hair and enormous blue eyes. Katrina did not acknowledge their presence, but stared right through them as if she was in a trance. She moved her arms around, reaching high above her head like she was trying to touch the sky. As they stood there, she opened her mouth and let out another piercing scream! It penetrated to Jan's soul.

Jan turned to the RN and asked if she could sit down and try to hold her. Miss Potter said, "Absolutely. But if she tries to get down, just let her go."

Jan walked over to a chair near the child, and moved it a bit closer. She sat there for a few minutes so Katrina would get used to her presence. Jan then reached over and touched one of her delicate little arms. Katrina did not move away, so Jan leaned down and gave her a light hug. To her amazement, she didn't resist. Jan then brought her up to her lap, and Katrina just sat there and continued to raise her arms and look vacantly out the window. As Jan held her, Katrina let out another scream, and Jan whispered, "It's alright, everything is going to be alright. You're such a pretty little girl. You have lovely hair and beautiful eyes." Jan continued to hold her while she rocked her gently. "We love you, Katrina."

After she put Katrina in her own chair, she asked Miss Potter, "Do students have access to the histories of the children?"

"Oh yes, and I encourage you to read about the children. Come and I'll show you the chart room." She then took them down to a little room behind the desk where the charts were kept. There was a long table in the center of the room with several chairs available. They sat down, anxious to know this precious little girl's history.

Kim began reading her history aloud, helping them to gain valuable insight into Katrina's background. "Katrina was rushed to the emergency room when she was three years old. The police were summoned to the neighborhood where she lived with her mother and countless males. A person living down the street was disturbed by Katrina's loud shrills. When the police arrived, they found her mother under the influence of heroin. Katrina was extremely emaciated and near death."

Kim's voice cracked with emotion, so Jan picked up the chart. "The patient was admitted to the Medical Center where she spent months on the pediatric ward for observation and countless diagnostic tests. They found extreme evidence of both sexual and physical abuse. There was so much physical damage to her little body, that they were forced to remove Katrina's uterus which was bruised and infected"

Jan's tears kept her from reading any further, so she passed it to Cindy. "Slowly her weight improved, but the emotional scars remained. A pediatric psychiatrist spent endless hours with her, trying to restore her mental condition. She appears to be in a static state of equilibrium and was released to the Watkins Home for custodial care. Diagnosis was 'semi-catatonic state' most likely permanent."

Cindy stopped to blow her nose and said, "I think we should take her to the dormitory so we can take turns nurturing her!" There would be many times the girls would feel this way while working in the Watkins Home. Jan decided to return downstairs and talk to Sandra again while Kim and Cindy went room to room observing. She came to Sandra's room and was surprised to see another RN working with one of the babies. She walked up, introducing herself. "Hi, I'm Miss Winston. Do you work here as well?"

"Yes I do. My name is Miss Chan, and I'm happy to meet you."

"Likewise. We were told there were only two RNs working here-one in charge of each floor-but you make three. Would you help me understand?"

"Absolutely. There are two RNs on each shift around the clock. Miss Ripley is the supervisor over all, and she only works during the day shift. She is the one we report to; however, I understand Miss Potter and I will be giving you students your assignments."

Jan thanked her and stood back to watch her work. Miss Chan was a beautiful lady with black hair cut short, expressive black eyes and a lovely smile. She reminded Jan of a china porcelain doll.

"When you have a minute, would it be possible for me to ask you a question in private?" Jan asked.

"No problem, I'm almost finished. If you could take this dirty linen over to the linen bag, I can finish up." Jan turned to start back as Miss Chan said, "Okay, we can step outside now."

"Could you explain what caused these children to have such large heads?"

"They have a condition called Hydrocephalus, which is a congenital defect that keeps the fluids from draining off the brain; it then accumulates excessive amounts of cerebrospinal fluid. Because the skull is pliable in a baby, it starts to expand and become very large. Sandra, though limited in her motor skills, is unusual for her ability to speak."

Jan asked, "What is the normal life expectancy?"

"Generally, just a few years. In fact, the next oldest has just turned five and will most likely die before he turns six. Sandra is the exception, she is eight."

"Isn't there anything that can be done for them?"

"So far medical science has not been able to come up with a fix. I personally don't think it will be too long before they find a way. Sad that it will be too late for these children."

"Thank you, Miss Chan. I'm going to visit Sandra and then go back upstairs."

Jan soon returned to second floor, and spent time looking here and there. While doing so, she found a nearly vacant room for play or some kind of activities. There were three boys in the room. Two were pushing toy trucks and another sat forlornly on the floor moving his head around in a rather bizarre manner. Jan sat on a couch to observe their behavior and the little boy about four years old got up off the floor and stood directly in front of her. He had very blond hair and a handsome face. She tried to talk to him, but all he did was sway back and forth making painting movements with his hands. She smiled while watching him even though he didn't smile back. He would not make direct eye contact. He looked everywhere but at her. Jan was about to get up when he surprised her by coming forward and crawled up on her lap. She put her arms around him for a hug, but he acted upset, so she let go. Out of the blue, he put both of his hands on her face and rubbed her cheeks up and down. Then he moved his hands to her hair smoothing the strands between the palms of his hands, still without any direct eye contact. He turned in her lap and played with her hands, making circles on her palms with his fingers. His touch was so light, it tickled, but she held still so he wouldn't leave. Next he faced her again and touched her breasts. She gently moved his hands to her arms, and he immediately went back to her chest, and this time he squeezed. Jan said, "Okay, you better get down," while gently sliding him off her lap.

As soon as his feet touched the floor he started to babble and swing his arms through the air, throwing his head from side to side. Jan wasn't sure what she should do when a caretaker came through the door and gently asked, "Is everything all right in here?"

Jan was about to explain when Mrs. Stewart flew in the door screaming in a high pitched voice, "Get out of this room immediately!" Her shrieking voice made the little boy go absolutely crazy, screaming and crying, turning around in circles and hitting his head with his hands. Jan wanted to scream at her instructor as she backed out of the room.

Mrs. Stewart gruffly said, "Come with me." The speed with which she walked made Jan feel like she was in a cross country ski race. Her instructor stopped at the desk and demanded a private room.

Miss Potter shot Jan an understanding look and pointed her finger behind her saying, "The chart room is empty."

Mrs. Stewart led the way and told Jan to take a seat at the table as she did the same directly across from her. She placed both hands on the table in front of her and stared at Jan with piercing black eyes "What in the world did you do to that child? I specifically told you to observe the children, not interact with them!" she shouted.

Jan had to strain to keep from screaming at her instructor. With a great deal of difficulty, she said in a calm voice, "I went into the room with the sole intention of observation. As I. . ."

Mrs. Stewart interrupted sarcastically, "I didn't ask you what you went in the room for, I asked what you did to that child." She slapped the table with both hands and screamed again, "Now tell me!"

Jan jumped in her chair and answered, "I'm trying to!"

The glare in Mrs. Stewart's eyes would have detonated an atomic bomb!

Jan continued emphatically, "As I sat there observing, the little boy climbed up in my lap and touched my face and hands, but when he touched my breasts and squeezed them, I slid him off my lap."

Mrs. Stewart fumed, "Was putting him in your lap a part of observing, Miss Winston?"

"I didn't put..."

"Don't get smart with me, young lady."

Jan wanted to say so many things, but knowing they would fall on deaf ears, she sat with her hands folded on the table and kept her mouth shut.

"Miss Winston, what is the definition of observe?"

"To watch."

"And did you?"

"I guess I should have thrown him to the floor when he crawled onto my lap?"

"That does it! Miss Winston, I will report your disobedience to Miss Kingston immediately. Now I want you to go out there and apologize to Miss Potter. Then return to this room until lunch."

Jan went out with Mrs. Stewart right on her heels. Jan said to Miss Potter, "I'm so sorry that I caused that little boy to react the way he did."

Miss Potter purposely glanced at Mrs. Stewart as she answered, "Miss Winston, you did nothing wrong. He has those kind of episodes throughout the day, but he does react far worse when there is screaming in the room." She shot an accusing look at Jan's instructor.

Jan smiled and asked Miss Potter if she could look at the boy's chart before lunch.

Miss Potter said, "Absolutely. His name is Wyatt Barr."

They had both ignored Mrs. Stewart. Jan turned to go into the chart room and as she awkwardly passed Mrs. Stewart, she glared at Jan before turning on her heel and stomping down the hall like a disgruntled teenager.

Jan found his chart and immediately went to his diagnosis: Aspersers Syndrome with psychoses, a facet of Autism. As she read his history, it was obvious that at a young age his parents had noticed something different about him, and their pediatrician had recommended removal from the home to be placed with children "of his kind." Jan wondered how difficult it would have been for his parents and if he had felt abandoned by them.

Cindy and Kim stopped at the door and said, "Miss Winston, it's time to go to lunch."

She pushed past them, hollering thanks as she ran out, down the middle courtyard, through the med center, and down the front stairs to the dorm. She waved at Allen who was patiently waiting, leaning on the passenger side of his car, as she ran in to change her clothes for college classes.

CHAPTER SIXTEEN
CAROL TO THE RESCUE

She greeted Allen with a sweet kiss. "Did you run all the way?"

She laughed and answered, "Sure. It would take me way too long if I just walked."

"Okay. Tell me about your morning, I can't wait to hear about it."

Jan revealed the details of her morning with Mrs. Stewart. Her anger escalated as she spoke. Allen listened attentively..

"It sounds like you have a severe mental case on your hands. How in the world did she get this job?"

"I wish I knew."

Allen pulled into a large park that was close to the campus. With a twinkle in his eye, he said, "I have a treat in store for you." He parked and got a couple of large paper bags and a blanket from the trunk , "Come on, there's a shady spot right over there." He put down the blanket and set out sandwiches, chips and a couple of root beers. Jan was thrilled because now she didn't have to be careful what she said in this isolated spot. She continued with her story until Allen stopped her, saying, "What is this woman doing as a nurse, let alone an instructor? Did she come out of the Dark Ages?"

"We're wondering the same thing. She displays no compassion whatsoever with those darling children. This is my first experience with her other than in the classroom, and I am really considering going to Miss Kingston about her. Do you think I dare?"

Allen thought for a minute and said, "Why don't you wait for awhile, and all three of you observe her actions around the children. You can also watch how the RNs react to her, and maybe get them involved. Then it wouldn't be just you."

"Well I know already how Miss Potter feels about her. I think she was about ready to strangle her! I know she heard the way Mrs. Stewart treated me in the charting room and it was obvious she didn't like it."

"Good. Sounds like a plan. Now let's get on with a more important topic, like us."

Since they were very much alone and surrounded by trees, he put his arm around her, bringing her down on the blanket in his embrace, kissing her with the same intensity of their first kiss. He pulled back, looking at her with a kind of love she had never dreamed of. He kissed her again. She completely lost her voice, overcome with emotion.

He continued to hold her close as he said, "Do you believe in God?"

"You know I do."

"I believe that God brought us together as part of His plan, and we were a match made in heaven. What do you think?"

Jan could hardly catch her breath, the magnetism was so strong between them. She sat up to breathe. "Absolutely. How else can I explain these feelings?"

"We need to pursue this subject further, but we'd better eat before it's time to go to class again."

They finished their sandwiches, then Allen reached to pick up their things.

"Wait. I need to tell you about something that happened to me about three years ago."

"Can you tell me on the way to our classes?'

"Not really. I need more time to talk about it."

"Okay. How about later?"

"Sure."

* * *

The next morning Jan returned to the Watkins Home. She found it fascinating to work with these children. Mrs. Stewart started them out in the morning, then promptly left --- to everyone's enjoyment. The only drawback was, they didn't know when she would pop in.

Jan, Kim and Cindy were assigned to help feed some children their breakfast in the dining room. The caretakers told them to hold the children's hands so they wouldn't play in their food. This really bothered Jan, but she went along with it since they had to follow orders. She fed three different children then cleaned them up afterward. She recognized many of the children as having Down's Syndrome. They were delightful, so happy and loving. Why in the world couldn't they function in their own family environment? She just didn't understand.

They walked down to Miss Ripley and asked, "Which floor do you want us to work on?" Miss Ripley looked up like she had no clue what we were asking or who we were.

"Ah, you and the dark-haired one, go upstairs. Then she pointed to Cindy. You stay down here."

Jan and Kim went upstairs to Miss Potter, and Cindy stayed with Miss Chan. Miss Potter was happy to see them and assigned one room for each with a caretaker to assist them.

Jan was delighted to be in the same room with Wyatt and quite a few other children much like him, as well as some with Down's Syndrome. She introduced herself to the caretaker. "Hi, I'm Miss Winston, and I'm assigned to work with you today."

"Of course, I remember you from the freak show yesterday with your instructor. I'm Carol, but I guess you're required to call me Miss Haven."

"Yes, those are the rules." Jan took an immediate liking to Carol, maybe because she was built so much like Mandy, a natural blonde with green eyes, and a special way about her that immediately put Jan at ease. She remembered her as the caretaker who had rushed in during the incident with Wyatt yesterday.

Jan learned immediately that these children responded most to patience and gentleness. She observed Carol and was impressed with her loving mannerisms. She knew she could not rush these children or discipline them harshly. She spoke softly in terms they could understand.

After they finished the morning care, Jan asked Carol, "Could I talk to you about the incident with Wyatt yesterday?" They walked to the back of the room and sat down on a couple of chairs. Jan said, "I guess I should explain what happened before you came to the door."

"Yes, that would be helpful."

"I went in to just observe their behavior when Wyatt came over and crawled onto my lap. I didn't feel it appropriate to push him off, so I let him stay."

"That's absolutely right. It would have upset him if you had."

"He played with my face and my hands, and then he touched my breasts. I wasn't sure how to react, but when he squeezed, I gently slid him off my lap. That's when he started to get upset."

Carol had a sweet smile on her face as she said, "First of all, you have to realize that he has no concept of so called private areas. To him, breasts are no different than feet or hands, so he wasn't doing something that he knew was wrong. Now when an autistic child does something like this, it is up to the individual's comfort zone just where you want to draw the line. I personally don't think that your reaction was inappropriate. Since I was there when your instructor entered the room, I have another opinion about her actions."

"Quite frankly, Carol, I was completely shocked, and I watched how it compounded his reaction."

"The way Wyatt reacted is normal for autistic children, as you have seen some of the examples this morning. Keep in mind that the only time to discipline these children would be to prevent them from hurting themselves or others, which does not happen very often. They are seldom combative unless frightened or hollered at. You saw that example yesterday, and even then, he took it out on his own body."

Jan asked, "How do you know all these things? Did you learn from experience or did you go to school?"

Carol smiled, "Actually, I did learn much of this through trial and error, but I have to admit that I'm in college working towards my degree in social work."

"Wow, I'm really impressed. Do you work full time?"

"No, I work two days a week and weekends. I was here yesterday filling in for someone who called in sick. My normal days are Tuesdays, Thursdays, Saturdays and Sundays. That's the only way I can support myself."

"I really admire you for what you're doing. You are going to be a great social worker."

Just then, they heard a scolding down the hall from Mrs. Stewart, and Jan thought *Oh no, it must be Kim.*

Carol said, "You better be busy with the children. Why don't you go talk with Wyatt. He may not respond, but I sincerely believe he understands."

Jan went over to him just in time to see Mrs. Stewart enter the room. She walked up to Jan and said, "Show me the children you cared for this morning, and let me see their beds."

Jan walked around showing her, and just when she thought she was doing fine, Mrs. Stewart found a sheet and blanket draped onto the floor. Jan knew, without a doubt she had made the bed properly, but she also knew that Mrs. Stewart would jump all over her. Just as she predicted, Mrs. Stewart gave her a disapproving look and in a loud voice said, "Well I see that you forgot this one!" The children became restless at the sound of her shrill voice.

Before Jan could say anything, Carol walked up and confronted Mrs. Stewart with a quiet but stern voice saying, "I checked each of her beds when she finished, and they were perfect. Did you stop to think that one of the children might have pulled the covers out? And by the way, I do not appreciate your tone of voice disturbing my children!"

Mrs. Stewart steamed as she retorted, "I could have your job for talking to me that way!"

Carol snickered and said, "Be my guest."

Mrs. Stewart turned on her heel and stomped down the hall.

Jan turned to Carol. "Thank you for coming to my rescue."

As it approached lunchtime, Jan looked for Kim. She found her sitting with her back to the door, holding one of the little girls with Down's Syndrome. She watched for just a few minutes and heard Kim singing a sweet little song to her. While she watched, two other girls came over and quietly sat at her feet, listening to her sing. They had the sweetest smiles on their faces. It made Jan's heart swell. Kim started encouraging them to sing with her. They sang "I am a child of God and He has sent me here." Jan glanced over to see two caretakers leaning against the wall watching the sweet interaction between Kim and the girls. Jan hated to interrupt, but she saw Cindy coming down the hall, so she told Kim it was time to go. Kim hugged each of the girls, and they kissed her on the cheek.

As they left for lunch, Mrs. Stewart was nowhere to be seen. Cindy did tell them that she saw Mrs. Stewart come barreling down the stairs. She went directly to Miss Ripley and whispered something to her, then they disappeared into the chart room.

During lunch Cindy said, "I learned from Miss Chan what the houses behind the Watkins Home are used for."

Jan smiled at her. "Well, don't keep us in suspense. Tell us."

"They're used by employees of the children's home and the hospital staff who have no children. They live there rent free except utilities, and their salaries are slightly less to compensate for free housing. They can only be married if their spouse works here also.

"So, the mystery is solved!" said Jan.

CHAPTER SEVENTEEN
CINDY TELLS ALL

Jan didn't see Carol on the following Thursday and thought she might have been fired due to her standoff with Mrs. Stewart. That scared Jan so much, when she saw her on Saturday she gushed, "I'm so happy to see you."

"They can't get rid of me that easy." Carol told Jan. "They gave me the day off to compensate for the Monday I worked. I got a bit of a dressing down by Miss Ripley, but believe me, if Mrs. Stewart gives me reason enough to do it again, I will. She is completely insane!"

At lunch the girls talked about enlisting the RNs to help with Mrs. Stewart. Jan felt that they should wait a little longer, as Allen had suggested, with the possibility that Mrs. Stewart might actually hang herself.

Kim had a natural ability to nourish the children with love. She was blessed with a lovely singing voice and many children's stories locked in her pretty little brain.

"How do you know so many stories and songs, Kim? The children love you, and you have such a natural way with them."

Kim seemed surprised and said, "I learned a lot from babysitting, and one mother had a children's song book from her church that I memorized."

"Kim, have you thought about working with these children when we graduate?"

"Yeah, I have actually, but we'll see how it goes. To be completely honest, I don't think I could work here if the 'Dragon Lady' was still around."

"I know what you mean. What did she get mad about last week?"

"Oh, she said I was holding a child in my lap for too long."

"She doesn't have a clue what this place is all about, does she?"

"You've got that right."

Jan was learning so much about these children, regardless of Mrs. Stewart's disruptive behavior. She was convinced more and more that it just wasn't right to institutionalize these children. Yes, there were a few who likely could not be handled in a home setting due to severe psychoses, but they were by far a small minority. One day she broached the subject with Carol, who she knew would have the right prospective. Carol suggested that they talk a distance from the home where they couldn't be overheard.

They decided to meet at Carol's house behind the Watkins Home that evening. She said to bring along Kim and Cindy or anyone else that wanted to join in.

Jan asked Mandy if she wanted to come, but she said, "I have something I'm working on for Miss Page in surgery, so go ahead and have fun. I'll try to find Mrs. Stewart so she can join you."

"You do and you're history, Miss Mandy!"

It was warm enough, the girls could wear shorts and blouses. Carol made them feel completely at home and had a plate of warm cookies waiting. Carol said, "Feel free to voice anything you'd like to discuss."

Cindy popped up first, sitting on the edge of the seat of an over-stuffed couch. "After seeing these deformed and pitiful kids, I just can't believe there's a God anymore."

Jan was stunned but not really surprised by Cindy's comment. Carol made the first response. "Cindy, have you ever felt this way before?"

"Oh, yeah!"

"Do you want to talk about it?" Carol asked.

Cindy sighed and hesitated, "You sure what I tell you won't ever leave this room? I really mean it. I'm about to tell you something I've never told anyone before."

Jan said, "Absolutely, Cindy, you know you can trust us, we're members of the elite Watkins Home trio."

Kim spoke up, "Cross my heart and hope to die if I ever breath a word."

"Go ahead, honey. You're safe in my home." Carol added.

"I was five years old when my fifteen-year-old brother woke me very early in the morning and carried me into his room. He hurt me really bad."

Jan asked, "How did he hurt you?"

Cindy looked down at the floor and whispered, "You know."

Carol asked, "Honey, did he sexually hurt you?"

"He told me he would kill my mother if I told anyone. I ran away from home the next day. When I was found and brought home, I tried to tell my mom what happened. She slapped me with a damp wash rag and told me never to say such a thing like that again."

Carol moved over, sitting next to her as she put her hand on her shoulder, she said, "It's alright Cindy. We're here for you."

Cindy continued. "My mom told me that God would hate me for telling such a lie. I didn't know who else I could talk to, and I felt like I was the one who had done something wrong. I didn't think God would let something like that happen, so it was hard for me to believe there was a God!"

Carol gave Cindy a hug while she gestured to get some toilet paper so Cindy could blow her nose. While Cindy paused to blow her nose and regain her composure, Carol asked, "Have you ever felt like you could believe in God again?"

"Yeah, in high school I had a really good friend who was a lot like Jan and Kim. She went to church every Sunday and she invited me to some of their youth activities. I even dated her brother for a while. He was a really decent guy. They made me feel good about myself, so I started to go to church with them. My mother was mad and upset when she found out and wouldn't let me see them anymore. I would still hang out with them at school, but then something really, really bad happened." Cindy started to sob and could hardly catch her breath.

Carol rubbed Cindy's shoulders saying, "It's alright honey. Just take your time."

Cindy struggled awhile before she found her voice. "They were both killed by a drunk driver in a head-on collision. Why would God let something like that happen?" Tears ran down her face. "Now I see these pitiful, confused little children; I'm certain a kind and understanding God wouldn't do this to innocent children."

"Oh honey, I feel your pain," Carol implored, "I can understand why you feel that way, but I want you to know that I feel God's presence in and around these children every day They're not necessarily that way because of God. Many have problems because of something their parents did or didn't do. Look at poor little Katrina, for example. She was abused to the point of no return. But when you hold her and show her love, she feels it. Possibly she will come around someday. They have been making discoveries lately about certain vitamins that may play a role in the growth and development of the fetus. In fact, they think that the lack of them may easily play a role in birth defects. I truly believe that God is behind this research."

Jan moved over in front of Cindy, knelt on the floor, and took Cindy's hand in hers and said, "Cindy, I want you to know how much I love you and know that you are a very wonderful person. I also know God loves you, too. He loves all of his children, but He can't always stop them from making stupid mistakes, such as the drunk driver that killed your friends. He gave all of us the ability to make our own decisions. If He hadn't, the world would be a perfect place and there would be no way for us to learn on our own. Even then He tries to guide us with a little small voice which we don't always listen to, honey."

Cindy suddenly pulled away from them and became quite agitated, burying her head in her hands, rocking back and forth.

She moaned; her eyes filled with tears again, and as she looked at Jan, she blurted out, "Jan, I felt it! Oh my God, He was actually talking to me!"

Jan and Carol were frozen in a time warp, not sure how to approach this change in Cindy's behavior. Finally Jan said, "Tell us about it, Cindy. Go ahead. It's alright to tell us."

Cindy shook her head back and forth. Then, looking right into Jan's eyes she said, "When one of the surgeons, Dr. Worthington, invited me over to his home a few months ago while I was on my surgical rotation, I felt this gnawing feeling in my gut not to go. Something kept saying, 'Don't go. Don't go.' Oh, why didn't I listen? I went anyway because he really turned me on. Oh, Jan, I spent the night with him, then he dropped me like I was a used banana skin! I should have listened. I really should have listened! Do you think that voice was God talking to me? Do you really?"

Jan and Carol both said, "Absolutely."

Kim, who had been sitting very still, taking this all in, suddenly came over beside Jan on the floor and said to Cindy, "Honey, we don't always understand what God's motives are, but since you now have a concept of why He was warning you, it will help you to listen next time. We also don't have a clue why He brings these children into the world like this, but we have to trust that He has His reasons. I had a friend who became paralyzed from a fall off his bike on a mountain trail. After I saw him in the hospital, I asked my dad why God would let him be this way for the rest of his life. You know what Dad said? 'Maybe to help us learn by giving of ourselves in service to Him.' And that's what we are doing for these children. Look how it's helping us to grow."

Cindy sat quietly on the couch as we surrounded her in a blanket of love. She looked at each of us. "I think I'm starting to understand. You're all so good to me, letting me talk about these things."

Jan said, "You want to know a secret?"

Cindy asked, "You have a secret?"

"Well, sort of. Good ole Dr. Worthington came on to me too and I bet he does it to all the students."

Cindy looked at Jan and giggled, "He thinks he's a Casanova, doesn't he?" Her voice was still weak from emotion. Cindy asked, "Hey, Carol, do you have any milk to go with those cookies?"

"You betcha, sweetheart. Coming right up as soon as you clear a path for me."

They made small talk while they munched on cookies. Then Carol said, "Jan, you wanted to talk about something to do with the children."

"Oh, I almost forgot since something much more important came up," Jan said, smiling at Cindy. Well as I have been watching and learning from these children, it has occurred to me several times that they would be better off in a loving family environment. Why do doctors immediately recommend institutionalizing them instead of placing them in their own homes?"

Carol was now on the edge of her seat, "Oh, you have brought up one of my favorite subjects. Do you realize that doctors seldom set foot in the Watkins Home? Do you know 90% of doctors, to my knowledge, have never recommended keeping these children at home and they discourage parents from ever doing so? Do you know that doctors even discourage parents from coming here to see the place before or after admission? I have written letters to the American Medical Association about the matter and never even received an acknowledgment. This is going to be my main focus when I receive my degree, and I hope to get a job at this medical center. I will then be in the department to help counsel parents on this crucial decision. She wrung her hands together. Oh I am so going to enjoy doing that."

"So I take it you agree with my feelings on this?" Jan said facetiously. They all laughed.

Since they had Carol's undivided attention, Kim asked, "Why do we hold the children's hands when we feed them? Why not teach them how to feed themselves and save staff time?"

Before Carol could answer, Jan commented, "I agree. In fact, I would wager that at least 75% would be able to feed themselves. Sorry, Carol. I just had to add my two cents."

"Oh, you're okay, Jan. I couldn't agree more. When I first went to work there, I asked Miss Ripley if we could at least give them a try. Her reply was 'absolutely not!' I have observed Mrs. Stewart with Miss Ripley many times and it appears they feed off each others' negative attitudes towards these children.

"That reminds me," Jan asked, "Do you know if Mrs. Stewart and Miss Kingston are sisters?"

"Oh, yes, of course they are. They live together."

Jan had a quizzical look on her face and asked, "What's with the "Mrs." as in Stewart?"

"She was married years ago. Didn't last long, she kept the Mrs."

"Wow," said Jan. Guess that rules out reporting her actions to Miss Kingston."

"Not if you get some RNs involved."

Kim spoke up. "Do you think Miss Potter and Miss Chan would go for it?"

"Yeah, I do. They have seen enough to blow her socks off! But let me approach them first and get a vibe for their feelings about her and how much they are willing to risk talking to her, okay?"

"Sounds good. Guess we had better be on the run. Dorm doors are locked in ten minutes!"

They thanked Carol and hugged her goodbye. Then they took off running.

CHAPTER EIGHTEEN
(Late Spring 1959)

ALLEN HITS THE JACKPOT

Allen picked Jan up early Sunday morning, and they started on their way to see his folks. Jan felt so relaxed this time compared to the last trip they made. She talked about some of the things that were discussed at Carol's house, but she left out the personal issues about Cindy. She knew those were confidential. She needed to honor her promise even though she trusted Allen completely.

As they drove, they both got really quiet. Jan remembered how Allen had stopped so suddenly along this same road and had given her their first real kiss. Out of nowhere, Allen pulled over, stopped the car, ran around and pulled Jan out of the car. He wrapped his arms around her and when their lips met, it was with the same intense emotion all over again. She couldn't ever imagine kissing anyone else again. He pulled slightly away and said in a soft voice, "Oh, Pumpkin, I do love you!"

Jan could barely whisper, "And I love you, too!"

They kissed again and since no car honked it's horn, they kissed one more lingering time. Reluctantly, they got back into the car. Before Allen could drive away, Jan said, "Wait, Allen, I really need to talk to you."

"Sure," Allen said as he rolled down his window. "The floor is all yours."

"Allen, something very terrible happened to me a few years ago, and I need to tell you, but at the same time I'm scared."

"That sounds pretty serious, but don't you know by now you can tell me anything?"

"Yes, but this is something really bad and it's awfully hard for me to put voice to a hideous memory that I've tried very hard to forget." She hesitated.

"It's alright. Nothing you could say would keep me from loving you."

"Even if I told you I was raped by a horrible man?"

"Are you serious?"

"Yes, Allen. I wish it weren't true, but I'm very serious."

"Jan, no! That's terrible!" He ran his fingers through his hair and shook his head while staring out the front window. "I can't imagine what you must have gone through. Oh, Heaven forbid," he said with pain in his voice. He opened the door, muttering, "I need some air." He jumped out of the car like a jack rabbit afraid of his shadow.

Jan sat there quietly sobbing, thinking *I knew this would happen. No decent man would want me.* She felt like she was being smothered. *I need to get out of here!*

She threw open her door and began to run towards the road. She nearly reached it when she was picked up by familiar strong arms. He cradled her in his arms as he whispered in Jan's ear, "Why were you running away, Pumpkin?"

She struggled to get down, "It's okay. I always knew no man would want me! Let me go, I need to get away!"

Allen held her tight, carrying her back to the car as he said in a rough voice, "You're not going anywhere until we talk. Do you understand?"

"Okay, but it's useless. You don't have to stay around. I'll just go on with my life without you."

Allen snickered as he said, "Yeah, like I'm capable of living my life without you."

He sat her down in her seat. "You promise you're not going to bolt out of here while I go to the other side of the car?"

In a meek voice, Jan answered, "No. I'll stay."

After he was seated, he gave a long sigh. "Look, I'm sorry I got out of the car that way. I just had to catch my breath and think for a minute. Now, are you able to tell me what happened? Can you do that?"

"It's so painful. I don't know if I can handle it, and I really don't know if you can."

"You don't have to go into full detail; just give me the guy's name so I can kill him!"

"I don't remember his name, honestly; but I can tell you how it happened."

Jan relived the horror of that night as she replayed the scene for Allen. "It made me feel dirty and used, like no good man would ever want me after that." She sobbed.

Allen reached over, taking her in his embrace. "How could you think that, Pumpkin. You tried to stop him. You tried to get those idiot friends to help you. You did everything within your power and strength to keep him from his monstrous act. You must forgive yourself, sweetheart, and know it doesn't change anything between us."

"Are you sure?" She began to sob. "I mean, do you realize I'm no longer a virgin?"

"Jan, Pumpkin, it doesn't matter. You'll always be pure to me. All that matters is what's in your heart, and I know how innocent and perfect you are."

Jan looked at him, and all she could say was, "Thank you. You're so wonderful to me. I feel better now that I've been able to tell you. I was really afraid I would lose you if you knew."

"How could you ever think that of me? It would take a very shallow person to walk away from someone as wonderful as you because of that. But I know one thing. I'd hate to run into him on the street. I'm afraid I might end up in prison."

"Well, now that I've got red swollen eyes, do you think we'd better get on the road again?"

"Sure, guess we'd better."

Allen was quiet for awhile, letting everything sink in until he blurted, "This happened in San Francisco, right?"

"Yes. why?"

He ignored her question. "And it was at your professor's house?"

"Yes. Why do you want to know, Allen?"

"Because I want you to take me there so I can give him a piece of my mind!"

"Allen, I really don't want to revisit that place and pull the scab off the wound that I managed to heal a long time ago. Please don't ask me to do that. Please."

"I'm sorry. I didn't look at it from your point of view. Guess we better close the subject, okay?"

"I think that's a great idea, and thank you, Allen."

"By the way, something good may be happening with my dad. Mom said he's become unusually quiet lately, like he's deep in thought; and she hasn't seen him drink at all. She hopes it's some kind of sign that he may be changing, but only time will tell."

"Allen, I feel sorry for your dad. I think he has built this wall around himself, and he would like to change, but he has no idea how to break it down."

They fell silent again, keeping their thoughts to themselves as they drove. As they turned into the road to his house, Allen remarked, "Did I mention this is all my parents' property and the cattle and horses you see on each side are theirs also?"

"You're kidding. All the way to the house?"

"Yep. And that large hill behind the house too, but we can't use it for the animals because there are a whole lot of abandoned mine shafts up there."

"Mine shafts from what?"

"Gold mining-the hills are filled with them. I pretty much know where they are from exploring when I was a kid. Dad taught me how to identify the ones that small branches, leaves and grass have camouflaged the hole over the years. If you should stand on one by mistake, you would fall in from your weight. If you know what to look for, you can see a slight indentation in the ground that looks out of place."

"Has anyone ever fallen down one?"

"Not to my knowledge, but Dad and I found a dead deer one time at the bottom of one."

Just then they saw the house and his mom working with her flowers out front. When she heard the car, she stood up and gave them a big wave. She greeted Jan with a kiss and a hug before she greeted her son. They went into the house where something in the kitchen had filled the house with such a mouth-watering aroma that Jan's stomach started to rumble.

Allen's mom said, "Come into the kitchen. I put some munchies out to keep you from starving until our big meal is served. I'll try to have it ready soon so you can get an early start home. I know you both need to study."

Allen remarked, "Actually, Mom, we just started semester break so we can stay a little later. Of course, Jan has to be to work at the hospital early in the morning."

"Oh, that's a shame. You have to work, Jan? But you do get paid for it, don't you?"

"I really wish I did. Student nurses are free labor to the hospital for three years. Of course we do get free room and board, but on the other hand, our entry fee more than covers that."

"Oh my, that doesn't seem fair."

"You're right. Especially now that we'll be seniors next month. We do everything that the RN's do and we do it for free."

Allen looked at Jan and said, "That's okay, Pumpkin. They'll miss you when you're gone. Mom, are we going to be alone with you today?"

"I'm not really sure. Your dad didn't come home last night, but that's not unusual. Oh, that reminds me; after I told him that you and Jan would be up on Sunday, he brought me a large, taped-up box and said to be sure and give it to you whether he was here or not."

She went into her walk-in pantry, but before she would let her son pick it up, she said, "Now he left strict instructions. In fact, they're written all over the box in his scroll. You are not to open it until you are alone in your room with the door locked-you cannot share what is in it with anyone except your wife."

Allen took the box in his hands and turned to Jan with a smile and said, "Well I guess we better get married so I can share this with you. Turning to his mom, he quipped, "We have no secrets between us you know."

Jan giggled and said, "Graduation is only a year away."

Allen groaned, "That sounds like an eternity."

They had a great visit. Jan told his mom about many of her experiences at the hospital. The meal was fantastic and they were reluctant to leave his mom alone. "Oh, by the way, a few days ago Frank came home looking like he had been in a brawl. He had a black eye, a bruised shoulder and raw knuckles. He told me I should have seen the other guy."

They hugged and Allen said, "Mom, please call me as soon as you hear anything about Dad, promise?"

"Yes, I promise."

Jan and Allen talked all the way home. The box was not mentioned, but they both felt its ominous presence on the back seat. In fact, it looked like an unknown passenger filling up the back of his tiny Volkswagen car.

Allen let Jan off just before curfew, drove to his room and carried the box inside. He left the box in the middle of the floor. He was so tired he laid down on the top of his bed. He suddenly woke up at two in the morning filled with a desire to investigate the box. He sat in his only chair, and pulled it in front of him. He grabbed his pocket knife and slit open the tape. Just as he did, he remembered his dad's warning to lock his door. He jumped up, turned the key in the lock and went back to the box. What he saw made him sit straight up like a cobra about to strike. He stared in disbelief. The entire box was filled with bundles of thousand dollar bills! They were stacked in neat rows and as he took them out, he could see the stacks continued down to the bottom of the box. *I can't believe the enormous amount of cash. I wonder, "Did Dad rob a bank? Did he take it out of the money Mom needs? Did he kill somebody for it? Now my imagination has gone wild, I just hope the police don't break down my door and drag me off to jail.*

Allen got up, pacing around his room to clear his mind. *I need to concentrate on what I know are absolute truths about my dad. I know that even with his change of attitude, he still lives by the same basic principles. Dad has always been honest to a fault. Everything he does is done with great integrity. I know down deep he still loves me and Mom.* Allen said out loud, "I wish there was an explanation. Wait a minute, I didn't look at the bottom of the box. Could it be he put some explanation in first and then covered it up?" He systematically took out all of the packets, and there in the bottom was a neat manila envelope with Allen's name on it. His hands shook as he opened it and slid out several legal papers.

On top was a letter that his dad had written in his definitive own style. Allen sat back and started to read out loud.

"*My dear son,*

I am filled with grief over the cruel way I have taken out my misfortune on you and your dear, sweet mother. Neither of you have deserved this. If I make it through the next few days, I hope I will have the opportunity to make it up to you.

For years the father of the boy that I shot and killed has been doggedly harassing me. He has made threats many times over. I have mostly ignored them, but he came into town last week, staying with his brother and drinking together every night at one of the bars. A friend told me they were trying to organize an old fashioned lynching party. Last week I confronted him and called his bluff. He tried to rough me up and I laid him out in the middle of the street! I went right to the sheriff and told him the whole story. He told me to lay low for awhile and stay at home except for necessary business in town. He told me this guy has a history of violence and has been in and out of prison. We don't think he knows where I live, but I'm not taking any chances so I may not be present when you come up, but I will be nearby.

Son, this whole thing has really got me thinking and I have been so out of line. I don't blame you for joining the service. If I had been living with me, I would have left too. I want you to know that for the last two weeks I haven't had a drop to drink and that was why I had an unfair advantage over this raging drunk maniac! If you want any more information, your old buddy, the sheriff knows my whereabouts and he can fill you in on the details.

Now, to explain the money. For a very long time, I have been putting money away in some different types of investments. You will find a signed document by the local bank president that this is legitimate money and he helped me pack the box. Take the money and the document to the bank with this letter Keep the money in an account where you can have access to it for your education and to start your dental practice. This is what the money was intended for in the first place. Put the legal papers from the bank president and this letter in a safe deposit box. Your mother is well fixed and will never want for anything. You already know the entire ranch is willed to you upon our demise and your piece of property remains in your name only.

Your mother knows nothing about this and I would rather you keep it to yourself. The sheriff is watching this guy, hoping he will pull something to justify putting him away. Please don't try to take matters into your own hands. That would not satisfy anything.

I'm hoping this will all be wrapped up soon and I promise that I will make every effort to change my bad behavior. I love you son and I'm so very sorry.

Lovingly, your Father, Frank Morris

PS You had better marry that pretty little filly you brought home with you. And please apologize to her for the way I acted. I guess I'm a pretty obnoxious drunk."

* * *

Allen put the letter down, and all the emotions he had suffered over the last several years came out in drenching tears. "I wish he could have told me himself." Allen muttered. "Still, maybe it was easier for him this way." Allen took a deep breath and dropped to his knees, "Dear God, I'm so grateful for my dad's foresight, I hope someday soon I can thank him in person. Please keep him safe."

Allen now felt uncomfortable with all of this money in his room. He gathered it together and put it back in the box, applying tape to tightly seal it, then sat in his chair waiting for the sun to come up.

He awoke still sitting in the chair, took a shower and waited for the bank to open. After settling everything at the bank, Allen gave a hearty laugh as he recalled the astonished look on the bank president's face when the box was opened. With some cash he went to a jewelry store, then made reservations for two at a really nice restaurant for the following Saturday night. Allen picked out the booth he wanted and explained his plans. He stopped by a florist and ordered a dozen red roses to be sitting on the table when they arrived. Allen was so nervous, just thinking about it that he had to settle himself down before seeing Jan that afternoon.

Allen decided to keep his job at the gas station for pocket money to avoid using the funds his dad had given him. He and Jan went bowling that evening, laughing and having a great time being together.

"Allen, you seem preoccupied with something." Jan remarked.

"Everything's fine. Just a little worried about my dad. Mom still hasn't heard from or seen him since we were there. Now I suggest you concentrate on getting a few strikes, my lady."

Back at his room, he called his mom, "Have you heard anything?"

"Son, I haven't heard a thing, I'm really concerned. He's never been gone this long; usually it was just for a day or so." Allen could hear the fear vibrating through her voice.

"I'm sure he's okay, Mom. Call me if you hear anything. Use the phone number at the gas station, since I'm scheduled to work tomorrow until closing. Don't hesitate to call, okay?"

"Okay, Allen."

The next evening, he was busy filling a gas tank and washing the windshield when he heard the phone ring. The customer took his time paying so Allen was unable to get to the phone. On a hunch, he called his mom, and as soon as she picked up the phone, she frantically said, "Son, is that you?"

Allen answered as his heart skipped a beat, "Yes, Mom. What's happened?"

She could barely talk. "The sheriff was just here and told me he was concerned because he was unable to find your dad in his usual location. I had no idea what he was talking about, so I asked him what was going on. He didn't answer my question, but he asked if I had seen any strange vehicles around the property or if anyone had come to the door asking about Dad. I did tell him that I saw a beat up old pickup parked on the main road just past our road when I went grocery shopping Saturday. He thanked me and said I'd been very helpful. He also asked if he could walk around the property a little bit, and of course I said 'yes.' Son, do you have any idea what's going on? Do you think your dad is in some kind of trouble?"

Allen tried to reassure her. "Mom, I know he has done nothing wrong to be in any kind of trouble. I'll drive up tomorrow morning and see if I can get more information, okay?" He hung up the phone just as another couple of cars drove in. He kept busy until closing, trying to call Jan just before leaving. The line remained busy until curfew.

CHAPTER NINETEEN

LOST

The next morning Allen was up at first light, driving right to the sheriff's office. He walked in the door, "Hi Allen, the sheriff's in his office," a deputy said.

Allen started towards the office as others greeted him. He could tell by the looks on their faces, they knew why he was there. The sheriff opened his door, "Come on in Allen, I've been expecting you and I'm glad you're here." He greeted Allen with a smile that would light the bottom of a coal mine.

Sheriff Savio gave Allen's hand a firm shake, "It's sure good to see you, the last I heard about you was when you took off to join the Air Force."

"Have a chair Allen. I'm sorry you had to drive up under these circumstances."

"Good to see you too Pete, I'm really concerned about my dad."

Peter Savio took his seat behind the desk and ran his hand through his thick wavy black hair. His dark brown eyes showing grave concern, "Allen, I just wish I had some good news for you. I walked around your folks' property yesterday and I did find this." He opened a drawer of his desk and brought out a red handkerchief in an envelope that was folded and smelled like chloroform.

Allen felt weak in the knees, unable to find his voice as he realized the implications. The Sheriff spoke again, "Allen, I know this guy is no good, and now he's been seen with his brother, adding up to double trouble. I did check at his brother's house, and it looks like it's been abandoned. I had a crew out there going through everything and questioning the neighbors. They all said they hadn't seen either brother since Saturday, except one neighbor mentioned that he saw them leave late Saturday night with both their pick-ups loaded with stuff. We have issued warrants for their arrest, to be brought in for questioning as persons of interest."

"Persons of interest! Do you think my dad has been murdered?"

"I wish I could say 'no,' but that is obviously one of the possibilities."

"Oh, no! Pete, I'm not sure I can handle that."

"I'm really sorry, Allen. We don't know anything yet so it's just a matter of time before we find him alive, I hope."

"My dad sent me a letter saying he was hiding out close by. Do you know where he was going to sequester himself?"

"You know the small building to the left of the big barn that generally houses the tractors and some farm equipment?"

"Of course"

"Well, since it has a small room and bath for hired hands attached, he's been staying there. He said it has a great view of the house and the road into it. He could also see the field behind the barn. When I looked in there, I noticed it has double doors--- one in the front and one in the back for easy access to the tractors. It's possible one of them could have distracted him at the front while the other might have sneaked up from behind using the chloroform."

Allen thought for a minute and asked, "Where did you find that handkerchief?"

"It was on the ground behind the barn."

"Sheriff, did you look around the hill behind the house?"

"Yeah, I did, but it was getting dark, and I couldn't see real well. I'm sending some men out there today to make a thorough search."

"If it's all right with you, I'd like to join the search."

"That would be great, Allen."

"Sheriff, do you have any idea what set the boy's father off after so many years?"

"The only thing we could come up with that might be related is that another son of his was shot and killed by a security guard while robbing a bank about six months ago. The father started harassing the security guard until recently the poor guy dropped dead of a heart attack." It could be that he figured he might as well take it out on your dad!"

Allen blew out a big breath and said, "Wow, this guy really scares me. Thanks for your help; I better get out to my mom's. I still don't know how much I should tell her."

"I'm sure you'll come up with something."

Allen waved his arm and walked out the door. As he drove up the familiar roads, his mind spun like a high-speed washer. His emotions were so fragile he was afraid he would break down in front of his mother, and that's the last thing he wanted to do. He began to rationalize, *I don't have to tell Mom about the father of the boy that dad killed, not yet anyway. He recalled to mind the scene following the shooting and the boy's father making threats.*

As the house came into view, he braced himself. His mom threw open the door and rushed out, wrapping herself in his embrace. He held her for a minute and then asked, "Mom, have you heard anything?"

"No, son, I'm beside myself with worry!"

"Let's go inside and talk, Mom."

Once they got settled on the couch together, Allen took her hand in his, "Mom, I talked to the sheriff, and he is sending a crew out this afternoon to search the property looking for clues to his disappearance. Who knows? We might find him in that old mine shack at the top of the hill taking a snooze."

"Allen, you don't really think that, now, do you? Are you thinking that he might have tried to commit.." She stopped herself with a sob as her hand went up to her mouth.

"No, absolutely not. You and I both know that Dad would never do such a thing. That's way out of character for him."

"Well, he's been out of character for a good many years!"

"I know, Mom, but I know Dad wouldn't do that." He patted her on the back. "I think I'll go out for awhile so I can get a head start before the deputies get here, okay?"

"Of course, son. In the meantime, I'll cook up some food for you."

Allen hurried out the door, calculating in his mind that it had been between four and five days since his dad's disappearance. If he was close by, he would be in dire need of water. He ran back in the house and asked his mom to fill a canteen.

When he was outside he thought, *I think I'll work my way around the back of the property and then go up the hill checking for mine shafts.* When he reached the top, he saw the mine shack. *Let's see if there's anything in here.* The door creaked open as Allen hesitantly pulled on it, *nothing in here, it looks the same as when I was a kid.* Allen sat on the ground in the shade of the old building, catching his breath. *What would I do if I had the distorted minds of those brothers? What would be my choice if I wanted someone to suffer and die? The most logical scenario would have to be, drop him down a mine shaft. The thought makes my heart chill! Dad could have been down in one for many days now. Oh, Lord, if he is please let him be alive. It could also be they took him with them when they left town. There are at least six places with easy access to drop him off a cliff to a hidden canyon. I can't think of him as dead, I can't get a handle on it. I really feel like he's alive, and it's urgent we find him!*

Allen heard vehicles on the road and knew the deputies were coming. He was already half way down the hill when he heard their doors slam shut. He approached Pete, "Allen, you're just in time to help in planning our search."

A deputy turned, "Hey Allen, welcome."

Another shook his hand, "Glad you can join us."

Allen recognized a few retired deputies that knew his dad well. One slapped him on his back, "You're a sight for sore eyes, Allen. Good to see you."

Pete cleared his throat, "Our primary focus will be the mine diggings. I've drawn a rough graph of the hill, and I'm putting two men teams in the middle of each area between these imaginary lines." pointing to the map. The sheriff paused and looked at the group of men. "Each team will crisscross back and forth to cover the entire area. Be mindful of those mine shafts; and holler loud and clear if you find anything or need assistance. Any questions?"

Allen was teamed with Don, a retired deputy he knew well. As they traversed back and forth, they scoured every inch of the ground for clues. About half way up the hill, they sat down to take a break and drink some water while beads of sweat poured out of them in spite of cooler weather. Don started to talk about the good times he had with Allen's dad. He was most likely in his early sixties, bald with a white fringe that traveled around the back of his head from ear to ear. He had a broad smile and a ruddy complexion. At one point in their conversation, he turned to Allen and said, "We really have to find that old coot. I'm not ready to let him go yet."

Allen said, "I'm tired of just finding a few spent shell casings along the way, I'd much rather find my dad."

The two men continued their tedious search. They finally crested the top ridge and waited for the other teams to arrive. Allen was not completely satisfied with their efforts. Sitting down, Allen voiced his feelings, "You know Don, it may be crazy, but every time we passed a mine shaft, we called out, 'Frank, are you down there?' But some of those are over a 100 feet deep. We probably couldn't hear him if he did answer!"

Don rubbed the back of his neck. "You've got a good point there, son. What do you suggest?"

Several of the men had gathered around to listen.

"Actually, on the really deep ones, I think one of us should repel down to take a closer look. I mean, what if he's, uh, unconscious or something." Allen couldn't get himself to use the word "dead."

One of the men hollered, "Here comes the sheriff. Let's ask him."

Allen turned to Pete, "I think we need to take our search a step further, Pete."

"What do you have in mind Allen?"

"I propose we go back in our teams and one of us propel down to check the deeper shafts."

"That seems reasonable, a few of you men go down and get some ropes from the vehicles and we'll put Allen's idea in place."

This would be more time-consuming, but Allen felt much better doing something. He and Don started down the hill together. "Allen, since I'm the heavier of the two, I'll hold the rope and slowly lower you into the deeper shafts, okay?"

"Sure Don, let's do it."

Each time Allen was pulled up, he was more disillusioned and wondered if this was worth the effort. After three tries, Don needed a rest. "That's hard work, Allen. I'm feeling my age, pulling you up."

"Do you want to trade places?" Allen suggested.

"No, I'm fine now." Don lowered Allen into a fourth shaft.

Almost overcome with bone-chilling fear, he called out, "Dad, Dad? Are you in here?" No answer came back. Allen searched the shaft, feeling morbidly discouraged. *If my dad is at the bottom of one of these earthly cold coffins, I can't imagine his suffering nor his*

ability to have enough energy to survive. Maybe we should just give up and call off the search!
"Okay, Don, pull me up. He's not in here. "Don braced his feet to pull when a gunshot boomed and startled him into losing his grip on the rope. Allen slid down several feet before regaining his footing. "Don? Is everything okay up there?"

"Allen, I'm so sorry. That was a gunshot. It must have come from on the other side of the mountain. I don't see anything, but let's get you out of there."

"Don, it's okay. Kind of gave me a thrill. We better find out what the shot was for."

They took off to investigate and found one of the deputies holding a very large diamond head rattler.

Allen stepped back, "Whoa, what happened?"

"This guy decided he wanted to join the search, and when I told him he wasn't eligible, he tried to shoot me. So I let him have it with my revolver!"

Since everyone had responded to the gunshot, Sheriff Savio spoke up. "Anyone find anything of interest?"

Allen looked around and saw shaking of heads and low murmurs. He was about to say "Let's call it off," but something held him back, and instead he put another piece of gum in his mouth and rubbed his chin.

Pete said, "Let's get back to work."

Allen and Don started down the hill from the mine shack. Allen suddenly stopped as though in a trance.

Don said, "Hey what's the matter, Allen?"

Subconsciously Allen realized he must look strange as he stood there gathering his thoughts. He slowly said, "Something is bothering me."

"What's that?"

"I'm sorry, Don. It just dawned on me, that last mine shaft, the one we keep passing, just down the hill, doesn't look quite right. I think I'd like to go there first and look at it again."

"I'll go with you, son."

It wasn't very far down the hill, and Allen just stood there staring down at it. Don looked at him and said, "What is it Allen? It looks normal to me."

"Don, as long as I've been coming up this hill, this shaft has always had a false top to it. How come the debris is down at the bottom? Bring your flashlight over here; I'm going to try something."

Don came closer to the shaft with his flashlight in his hand.

"Just shine the light on those branches and leaves below."

Allen got down on his knees, cupped his hands around his mouth and hollered at the top of his lungs, "Dad, this is Allen. If you can hear me, try to move the debris on top of you. If you can talk, holler as loud as you can!" They both stared at the leaves while listening intently.

Don said to Allen, "The leaves moved. Did you see that? Praise be to God. They moved!"

Allen hollered again, "Dad, if you're down there, I'm coming down to get you, and we'll have you out in no time." He then added, "I love you, Dad!"

Don lowered Allen down into the shaft, hollering for some men to come, "Hey, give us a hand over here, we think we've found Frank!"

A few men responded carrying their ropes. "Here, help me tie this rope around my waist, then take me down to help Allen." They worked feverishly to remove twigs, dirt and leaves. Allen was watching closely when he suddenly saw his dad's boots. Just then another man lowered himself down to help. Frank had tape over his mouth and as they removed it, Allen could not tell for sure if he was alive or dead. They pulled away the debris but he couldn't see his dad's arms.

Someone hollered down, "Is he alive?"

Allen touched his dad's face, "Dad please open your eyes."

Frank slowly opened one eye half way. The three men gave a sigh of relief, and Allen wanted to fall to his knees and say, "Thank you God!"

Allen hollered, "He's alive! can we get help pulling him up?"

They lowered a stretcher on a rope. Two men lifted him onto the frame, tying a rope to the other side. Then one of them gave the high sign to pull him up with the stretcher so he could guide it to safety.

The deputy with Allen said, "There's one rope left Allen, you go on up so you can be with your dad."

"Thanks," Allen said as the men above brought him up in record speed.

Don walked over, putting his hand on Allen's shoulder and said, "Hallelujah!"

One of the men came up from the vehicles, and stopped to talk to Allen. "I informed your mom and used her phone to send for an ambulance. Then he looked around at everyone and said, "He is alive, isn't he?"

Don answered in a voice filled with despair, "Yes, but he's not in very good shape."

Allen walked over to his dad laying helpless on the stretcher. Apparently the brothers had tied his arms behind his back, and he was in excruciating pain from laying in that position since they threw him down the mine shaft. A deputy had removed the ties around his wrists, but he could not move his arms. One of the men gave him a few sips of water. Frank tried to talk, and just a raspy unintelligible whisper came out. His eyes were still only half open. When he saw his son again, he started to cry.

Allen reached down and lightly patted him on his chest so he wouldn't hurt him. In an emotional voice he stammered, "It's okay Dad. Everything's going to be fine. They'll get you to the hospital, and I'll bring Mom in to see you right away."

His dad let out a raspy moan and continued to sob. They gave him another sip of water.

Allen went down the hill behind the stretcher, and he could see his mom standing next to the ambulance, twisting a handkerchief. He ran ahead, putting his arms around her, "Mom, he's alive. His arms were tied behind him so he's in a lot of pain and he can barely talk."

"Allen, will he be alright?"

"Mom, we'll know a lot more when he sees the doctor. I'll drive you to the hospital as soon as I clean up a bit and call Jan." Allen went inside to take a quick shower and put on clean clothes. He checked the time and knew that Jan should be at the dorm. Allen was ecstatic when the phone actually rang and wasn't busy.

He heard someone answer "nurses dormitory." It was Jan's voice.

"Jan, is that you? It's Allen."

"Oh, Allen, I was hoping it would be you. Where are you?"

"I've been searching for my dad and found him at the bottom of a mine shaft."

She sucked in a breath. "Oh, no. How terrible. Was it an accident?"

"No. Some bad guys tried to murder him. I haven't time to talk now. I have to rush to the hospital. If I'm able to get home from the hospital before your curfew, I will call you again and go into more detail."

"That's okay. Just take care of your mom and give her my love."

"One more thing. Reserve Saturday evening for a fancy dinner with me. Okay?"

"Okay. Do I need to dress up?"

"Well, I'm going to wear my suit."

"Oh, my goodness. What's the special occasion?"

"You'll find out Saturday night, Pick you up at six, okay?"

"Of course. I can hardly wait!"

"Me, too!"

Allen flew out the door and saw his mom waiting beside her car, holding the keys out for him. "Now Allen, I want you to tell me everything."

"Mom, the father of the kid that Dad shot years ago teamed up with his brother and wanted to kill Dad."

"No. After all these years, I had no idea. Have they caught those men yet?"

"I'm afraid not, but the Sheriff is working on it."

When they arrived at the hospital, they saw police cars everywhere. Inside, the waiting room was filled with deputies, wanting to know what the outcome would be. Pete immediately got up and gave Carmela Morris a hug, and then shook Allen's hand. "I've put an All Points Bulletin out on the brothers for attempted murder. I think we got them this time."

Just then, the doctor came out, and as he looked around the room, he said, "My goodness, who's watching the shop?" He turned to Mom and said, "Mrs. Morris, I'm sending Frank over to x-ray to see what the damage is to those shoulders. We are cleaning him up. He has an IV going to replenish his fluids. We'll need to admit him for observation. You can see him when he gets back to his room." He stopped, looked around and added, "Just his wife and son, okay men?"

The sheriff spoke up and said, "I really need a statement from him as soon as possible."

The doctor looked at him and said, "Okay, Pete, a brief one. I don't want him using his voice too much. Come on back with me."

Allen looked at his mom and said, "I just realized I'm really hungry."

One of the deputies popped up and said, "Don't worry about it, Allen. I'll just run down to Andy's Grill and have my girlfriend wrap up a nice meal for you and be right back. How about you, Mrs. Morris?"

Carmela looked at him and responded, "Oh heavens no, I couldn't eat right now, even if you offered me a free trip to Italy."

He was back in no time, and Allen scarped it right down. The deputy wouldn't accept a dime from Allen saying, "It was on the house when Andy found out who it was for."

Now he and his mom had to sit and wait for the final decision from the doctor. As they waited, Allen and the deputies talked a great deal about the harassment his dad had endured for a very long time. His mother sat listening; every so often Allen saw her wipe a stray tear from her eyes.

When there was a lull, she leaned over to Allen and asked, "Why didn't you tell me about this?"

"Mom, I just found out about it Sunday night when I opened the box and read the letter that Dad had enclosed."

"He told you all of this, and you didn't tell me when you got here this morning?"

"No, I felt it would just add to your grief, mom."

"Oh I suppose you're right."

Just then the doctor approached with a scowl on his face.

CHAPTER TWENTY

A CHANGE OF HEART

Allen jumped to his feet even though the doctor's focus was on his mom. The doctor sat down beside her and gently took her hand as he spoke in a guarded voice, "Mrs. Morris, Frank has some extensive damage to his right shoulder and upper arm. He told me he remembers landing on that side and heard something crunch just before he passed out. It's definitely going to need surgery for some intensive repair work. His left arm is also damaged, but not as severe, so I'm recommending we try physical therapy first, and then we'll re-evaluate. I have called one of the best surgeons in the state, consulted with him, and he's agreed to do the surgery next Monday. We both agreed we want Frank to be a little more stabilized before transporting him to the Watkins Medical Center."

"Oh my gosh, that's where my girlfriend is a student nurse. And it's the city where we both go to college. Wow, this is great!"

"Well, I seldom get that kind of a reaction to a loved one facing surgery. Nevertheless, it sounds like it will work out quite well for you. He's back in his room now, so you can see him. I have him heavily sedated temporarily so he can rest. He'll remain here until Sunday when the ambulance will transfer him down to the city. Do you have any questions?"

With her hand on the doctor's arm, Allen's mother asked, "Is he going to be all right, doctor?"

"He was severely dehydrated, which will take a few days to hydrate him. Other than his shoulders, it doesn't look like he has any other complications. We will be watching him closely for the next few days, and even though it may take a few months, I believe you'll have your husband back to normal before too long. Go to his room for awhile, and then I think you both need a good night's rest."

Allen took his mom's hand in his, thanked the doctor, and walked quickly to his dad's room. As predicted, his dad was sound asleep and nothing disturbed him. They talked about their plans. She would call her sister-in-law that lived in a suburb of San Francisco to see if she could stay with her. His mom turned to Allen, "I can probably follow the ambulance down in my own car and you can meet us at the hospital on Sunday."

"Mom, That sounds great, but right now I'm really tired. I'll go home with you and get a good nights' rest. I can talk to dad in the morning and get back in time for work."

"Not much reason for me to stay either. I put a pot roast and vegetables on this morning. It most likely has fallen apart by now, just the way you like it."

"Let's go."

It was too late to call Jan, so after a meal of his mom's home cooking, he fell into a relaxed sleep in the familiar surroundings of his old room and bed. The next morning they drove their own cars to the hospital so Allen could leave after visiting with his dad.

They walked in to an empty bed and a young nurse busily remaking it with clean sheets. She perked her head up. "Hi. The orderly took him downstairs for more x-rays, but he should be back any minute."

His mom immediately asked, "How is he this morning, dear?"

The nurse walked over to them, openly exhibiting interest in Allen. "Actually, I know he is in a lot of pain, but he asked that his shot be given after his family visited. He told me he didn't want to be 'drugged up' before his wife and son came in." She couldn't take her flirtatious eyes off Allen, touching his arm and fluttering her eyelashes as she spoke. "I'm sure he'll be back soon."

With an amused chuckle, his mom answered, "Thank you so much. You can go back to work now, honey," as she waved her hand towards the bed.

Just then they heard a raspy but familiar voice behind them saying, "Oh good, you're both here. I can hardly wait to visit with you."

They turned to greet Dad; Mom reached down to give him a quick kiss. He was not able to shake hands, but he started to cry when Allen stroked his back. His attention went to his nurse, "Help me into bed, sweetheart, and then I would like to be alone with my family for awhile." He sounded like a frog with a wire toothbrush stuck in his throat.

Allen and his mom stood watching as his dad winced in pain with the slightest movement. They moved to his bedside as the nurse left the room. "Can you ever forgive me for the way I've treated you?" His eyes glistened as he struggled to speak clearly. "They left me for dead, you know. Their intention was for me to die a slow, agonizing death. I figured I deserved it after the way I've acted for so many years."

Allen started to say something, and his dad shook his head to stop him, "I had a lot of time to think, and I suffered in anguish as I realized that your memories of me would be that terrible person that I had become. After the shooting incident, I became wrapped up in a shroud of self-pity until I could no longer see daylight. I hated myself day and night, and then I turned to the bottle to anesthetize my pain, which just intensified my bad behavior. I don't know how either of you can ever love me again."

Allen and his mom both whispered between their own tears. They had never stopped loving him.

He paused a bit, "Carmela, can you wipe the tears from my eyes and nose? I laid there in the bottom of that mine, shivering from the cold in that musty damp atmosphere, covered with leaves, dirt and branches that poked me if I moved, thinking that my destiny was to die in that hole and never be found. It was about the fourth day I think, when I would have paid anything for a drink of water and decided to make a deal with God." Between sobs he continued. "I told Him if He would allow me to be found, I would do everything possible to make it up to my wife and son and never go back to that horrible stranger again. It was some time later when I heard your voice, Allen, and I knew beyond any doubt He answered my prayer!" With a sob he concluded. "I just hope and pray you can forgive me, please!"

Allen could barely see through his tears as he said, "Dad, I love you with all my heart, and I have never stopped loving you. I didn't like what you had become, but you never lost my love, and of course I forgive you. Now you need to concentrate on getting yourself back in shape so we can go to the cabin again, okay? And Dad, I really appreciate the letter and the contents of the box."

"You're welcome, son. That's so you can make the name of Morris famous in your dental practice," he said with a sniffle.

"I don't know about famous, but if you don't mind, I'm going to leave you and mom alone. I know that you have a lot to talk about, and I need to get back to that pretty little filly you mentioned in your letter. I do love you dad, and I'll see you on Sunday, okay?"

"Whatever you say, son, and thank you again."

Allen walked out reeling from his dad's conversation. *Could it be? Was it real? Did he really have his dad back?*

As he drove back he thought, *I will be cautiously optimistic about Dad changing; realizing he may fall back into his old habits. Only time will tell.*

"Hi Larry, I'm back in town and ready to make up for time lost at work."

"How's your dad?"

"He's holding his own. They're bringing him down here for surgery and physical therapy on Sunday."

"Great. Listen, I need a couple of days off. Can you work Thursday and Friday for me, and I'll give you the weekend off?"

"Sure, no problem as long as I've Saturday evening and Sunday off, we're good."

"Okay. Thanks, Allen. Give my best to your dad."

Allen sighed as he hung up the phone, knowing this would stop him from seeing Jan until Saturday evening. He missed her so much he could hardly stand it. All he could do was wait until after her shift ended and then try to get through on the phone between his gas station customers.

* * *

It was Saturday morning when Jan, Kim and Cindy approached the Watkins Home with emotions in high gear. Kim said, "I can't believe this is our last day with the children, and to top it off, we'll be going our separate ways to new rotations next week."

"I know, I've gotten so close to both of you, I don't look forward to leaving." Cindy answered.

Jan observed, "We three have a bond that can't be broken and we'll always be friends."

When they entered the building, Miss Chan approached them. "Hello nurses," she said as she gave each a hug. Since this is your last day, your assignment is to spend some quality time with those children you've become close to. Does that sound okay to you?"

"Oh yes, thank you, thank you," they said.

Jan headed for the stairs and almost ran to Wyatt's room. She had made a personal connection with the autistic and Down syndrome children, but Wyatt remained her favorite. Jan greeted Carol with a hug, "You know today's our last day, so I will be spending some time with you," she said as she helped Carol tuck the linens in under a mattress.

"You can spend as much time as you want in here, I always enjoy your company." Carol said as she worked. "I consider you one of my best friends, Miss Winston."

"The feeling is mutual." Jan answered as she walked towards Wyatt. "Hello, Charlie and Wyatt. Hi there, Bobby." She could tell they were aware of her presence in spite of having little or no direct eye contact. Wyatt had been working his way toward her from across the room along with a few of the others. "Look what I have." Jan opened a bag that held some coloring books and crayons she purchased on her own. "Would you like to color with me?" She said while moving across the hall to the playroom.

One by one, four of the children followed her in and sat at the table with her. "It's fun to color, isn't it. There are all kinds of pictures, see?" She held the books up for them to see. She watched the children interact with each other, as they became intent with the process of using different colors in the books, for the most part repeating the same movements on a page.

Jan tried a little experiment. "Oh what a pretty picture of Cinderella. Let's see, what colors shall I use?" Wyatt leaned in closer to see. "Red would be pretty, I'll color her dress red. Okay?" Wyatt and another little boy watched her picture came to life.

Wyatt pushed his coloring book over to her and said, "Wyatt's?"

"I would love to color a picture for you, Wyatt. You pick out the picture you want me to color." She started turning pages until he pointed to one.

Wyatt held the coloring crayons, "This one." He handed Jan one at a time saying, "Mine." She finished and handed it back to Wyatt. "Do you like the picture, Wyatt?"

He looked right at her and said, "Keep?"

"Yes, Wyatt. You keep it."

Jan was filled with emotion as she moved to the couch. Two of the boys followed, Wyatt being one of them. He crawled up on her lap, and the other sat next to her. This time Wyatt curled up in a fetal position and allowed Jan to hold him close like she would hold a baby. The other child laid his head on her shoulder and curled up next to her. Jan was near to tears while they stayed in that position for about ten minutes. Carol came to the door and quietly said, "Before you leave, I need to tell you something."

The boys immediately got up and followed Carol out of the room. Jan went to Carol and asked, "What do you have to tell me?"

"We can't talk here. How about coming over to my place this evening and we can visit?"

"Oh, Carol, Allen has invited me for a date at a fancy restaurant. I can't tonight."

"That's okay. How about tomorrow?"

Jan laughed and answered, "We are going to be with his mom and dad tomorrow when they arrive at the med center so we can visit before his dad's surgery on Monday."

Carol answered with a look of concern, "My goodness, what's happened to his dad?"

Jan gave her a quick rundown then said, "Allen hasn't been able to tell me the details. His calls have been short-circuited between serving customers at the station where he works. I haven't seen him since last Monday because of his dad."

Carol looked at Jan with a whimsical grin, saying, "Then would you please check your calendar, Miss Winston, and tell me when you can work me into your busy schedule?"

Laughing Jan said, "Sure, how about Monday evening?"

"Are you sure you can be without Allen for one evening? And by the way, I need to meet this young man and give my stamp of approval."

"Sure, but he's working that evening and I'm not sure about the rest of the week."

"Okay, okay, I get the picture. See you Monday."

"Sounds good."

Jan walked down to find Kim and found her with Katrina in her lap. Kim was singing, "Teach me, guide me, walk beside me, help me find the way." Jan stood there watching, wishing she had her camera to capture this very special moment. Katrina was cuddled in Kim's lap, not making a sound, her arms wrapped around Kim's waist. Kim looked up, smiled at Jan and continued her singing. As she watched Kim and Katrina, her thoughts took her back to Katrina's screams. *It's been a few weeks since I've heard her scream. I think Kim has performed a miracle here. I wish I could go over and hug them, but I wouldn't dare break the spell! It's so wonderful just to stand here and watch.*

Jan walked down to the rooms that were filled with the Down's Syndrome children. She was immediately surrounded by happy hugs and kisses. *What beautiful children they are. It makes me sad knowing the parents of these wonderful children have been denied the special love these youngsters could have provided in their homes.* She spent some time in both rooms telling them stories and laughing together, first with the girls and then with the boys. They all gave her a warm send off.

Jan visited each room, purposely ending the day with Sandra. She loved this courageous little girl beyond measure. Oh, how she wished there was some way to fix this problem at birth so they would not have to suffer in heroic silence. She was able to have a quiet conversation with Sandra, feeling a measure of intelligence beyond her years.

"I'm going to miss your visits, Miss Winston, but don't worry; my mother has told me my time on earth is coming to a close," said Sandra

"Has your mother come to visit you, honey?"

"Not in person, she hasn't."

"I'm not sure I know what you mean, Sandra."

Sandra answered with a twinkle in her eye. "No Jan, she died following my birth."

How did I miss that in her chart? "Has she visited you often?"

"Oh yes, but the visits are more often now and sometimes she lays down beside me while I sleep. She's my guardian angel, you know."

Jan felt tears rising to the surface that she could no longer hold back. "Sweetheart, I'm so happy to hear you've had loving guidance from your mother, and I'm sure she's looking forward to being with you again. Just remember, I will always remember you and hold you close to my heart."

"Maybe I can become your guardian angel."

"That would be wonderful, honey." Jan leaned down and gave her a big hug, grateful that Mrs. Stewart was nowhere to be found. She pulled up the side of the crib and went straight to the chart room.

As Jan read her chart, she kept looking for some evidence of her mother's death and couldn't find it anywhere, not even in her history. Then at the very bottom of the chart, someone had folded a copy of Sandra's birth certificate and stuck it way underneath. Jan struggled a bit to pull it out, opened it and there beside her mother's name was a notation-"Deceased during childbirth." Jan let out a sigh, leaving it unfolded, and slid it in under "Important Documents." There, that's where it should have been instead of shoved in back like worthless trash!

It was time for the girls to leave. They had said their goodbyes and walked out the door hand in hand. Kim couldn't stop crying, "I'm going to return every Sunday to sing to Katrina. I love her so much, I would adopt her if I could."

"I'm going to miss the children and the friendships I've developed." Jan said.

Cindy concluded, "I can't stand the thought of being separated from the two of you. I'm really going to miss working with you. Please tell me we'll be friends forever."

Kim said, "Forever."

Jan added, "And ever."

CHAPTER TWENTY ONE
(1959)

ROMANCE IS IN THE AIR

Jan could hardly wait to get to her dorm room; she was filled with excitement about her formal date with Allen. She felt like she hadn't seen him forever even though it had been just last Monday. So much had happened since then, and they would have a lot of catching up to do. Allen had told Jan briefly about his dad, but there were so many questions left unanswered regarding his condition.

She went to her closet, looked through her dresses to see which one to wear. She decided on her light-weight, baby blue suit that matched her eyes and showed off her figure. She retrieved her white high heels from the back of her closet, and reached up to the shelf to pull out her matching white purse. She looked at the combination and called Mandy from down the hall to get her opinion.

Mandy took it all in, giving her approval as she turned to Jan. "You better get yourself into the shower. I'll help you put your hair in pin curls and they'll have time to dry.

Jan looked at her. "You are the best friend I've ever had."

"You can say that again. Now, go!"

Jan stuffed her uniform in her laundry bag, took her shower and when she returned, Mandy was waiting to do her hair.

When Mandy had finished, she said, "Now I'll do your nails while your hair dries. Pick a color Miss Winston."

Jan picked a pale pink and let Mandy do her thing.

"Mandy, you would have done well as a cosmetologist. It seems so natural for you. Why did you chose to be a nurse instead?"

"My mother wanted me to go a long way from home, and choose a career that would allow me to be self- sufficient. She knew I had the intelligence to go to college."

"Really, my parents told me I couldn't be an actress and made me choose either nursing or teaching."

Mandy giggled. "You wanted to be an actress? Oh, you would have been another Elizabeth Taylor-so beautiful and dramatic!"

Jan laughed out loud. "Me, beautiful? I know what I look like in the mirror, you know."

Mandy got really quiet, taking in a deep breath and seriously answered, "You must look with blinders on. Look at yourself, Janet Winston; you're beautiful even without any make-up."

Jan met her gaze in the mirror. "Like I said before, you really are my best friend ever and thank you. Now finish my nails, madam, or I won't give you a tip."

They both laughed, knowing deep down they had just exchanged something very special.

She was ready thirty minutes early. Jan went downstairs to their living room area, "My goodness, why is everybody gathered in here?"

"Waiting for you." "Jan, you're stunning." "I think she's a knockout." were some of the comments she heard.

"You can blame it all on Mandy; she tried to make me look like Elizabeth Taylor."

Mandy gave her a delighted smile as Jan sat in the chair beside her.

Never in her life had time dragged by so slowly. When the doorbell rang, Jan jumped. Cindy ran to answer it while Mandy put her arm on Jan to keep her seated. Cindy brought Allen in and the girls took a sharp breath as he came around the corner. Jan was blown away at how handsome he looked in his chocolate brown suit, shirt and tie to match. He was obviously embarrassed, but when his searching eyes found Jan, he murmured, "You look so beautiful." The girls whooped and hollered as she walked across the room, he took her hand and walked her out the door.

When they were settled in the car, he murmured, "I've missed you so much, you have no idea."

"Oh, yes I do. I've missed you too!"

They talked about his dad all the way to the restaurant, and she was thrilled to hear about his improvement and his change in attitude.

"You know, Allen, I'm pleased he will be at the medical center for awhile and I'll be able to visit him often."

As they arrived at the restaurant, Jan noticed that Allen was obviously nervous. This made her heart leap into an area of her stomach awakening those nervous tap dancers again. She barely heard him ask the host about the reservations for Morris. They were ushered to a secluded booth with a dozen red roses in the middle of the table. For a minute she thought the roses came as part of the ambiance of the eating place, then she looked at the nearby booths. There were no roses, only a small candle in the center of each table.

"Where did the roses come from?"

He actually looked embarrassed. "They're from me."

"Oh, they're beautiful. Is this a special occasion?"

He cleared his throat and said, "The waiter is coming. We better look at the menu so we can order."

"I don't have to; I already know what I want."

"What's that?"

"Prime rib, medium rare, baked potato with everything on it and a side salad."

"That sounds good for me too."

The waiter arrived, As Allen ordered, Jan took in the atmosphere of the restaurant-exclusive paintings on the walls, neatly pleated brocade drapes with matching plush carpet.

When he finished they sat looking at each other, grateful there was no candle because it would have melted and ruined the elegant tablecloth.

Their waiter broke the spell. He wore a black tuxedo and delivered their food on a sterling silver tray. It was definitely an atmosphere for the rich and famous.

Allen broke the ice. "Catch me up on the children and Mrs. Stewart."

Jan related the happenings of their last day. "It's been so peaceful. The wicked witch hasn't been around for awhile."

"Maybe she flew off on her broom."

"Hopefully the broom lost its way and took her into outer darkness."

They continued to talk about his dad and more details regarding his near-death experience.

He noticed she had put down her fork and stopped eating. She seemed to be lost in thought as she kept her eyes glued on him. "Jan you can't live on so little food."

"I always eat like this. Haven't you noticed? Besides, I'm saving room for dessert."

At the mention of dessert, he hurriedly got up from the table and excused himself, leaving Jan suspicious of his every move. He gave a high sign to the waiter, then disappeared. Jan's stomach went into orbit. She was sure the tap dancers had added some bagpipes to their repertoire, and she was being consumed with their antics. Just as she thought she couldn't handle any more, Allen returned looking like he had one of the bagpipes stuck crosswise in his smile.

Allen sat down. "I took the liberty of ordering dessert-your favorite, okay?"

Jan looked at him, "Thank you."

Their table was cleared, and Jan noticed staff hovering close by. Were they on display in a storefront window? The other customers leaned forward watching them expectantly. The tap dancers had now been replaced by a diesel truck revving its engine.

Jan looked up and saw their waiter approaching with one large, hot fudge sundae and two long handled spoons. *How romantic to have just one sundae they could share.* The waiter placed it in front of her, and as the waiter backed away, Allen took his place, kneeling down on one knee beside her! He took her left hand in his and said, "Miss Janet Winston, I pledge my complete, overwhelming love to you and I would be honored if you would accept my proposal of marriage, to be known as my fiancée for the next year until we both graduate."

Jan looked at Allen the entire time as he said such beautiful heartfelt words, unaware of those watching. She pulled him up to sit beside her and said, "Yes, absolutely yes!" She put her arms around his neck and kissed him with salty tears running down her face.

Only then did she become aware of people clapping and whistling. Allen stayed sitting next to her. "Shall we eat our dessert?" he asked.

She reached for a spoon, and as she picked it up, she saw something shiny attached to the stem of the ice cream goblet. She took a better look and let out a gasp! Allen said, "Here, let me help you with that," as he untied it from the stem. He took her left hand in his, gently pushing it on to her ring finger. "This is my promise to you, that I will always love you and support you for the rest of our lives together."

They kissed again, and someone in the crowd said, "Your ice cream is melting!" They all laughed, and Jan took a spoonful of dessert and fed it to Allen. He did the same, and the crowd went wild.

As people started to thin out, some stopped by to make comments to them. Jan's nerves calmed down and she was able to get a better look at her ring in the brighter light. She turned to Allen. "It's so beautiful."

Allen smiled and kissed her again, saying, "Nothing could possibly equal the beauty of the special lady who's wearing it."

"Allen, you are so wonderful to me. How did I get so lucky?"

"Not luck my dear. We are meant to be together."

"I know, and you have made me so happy tonight. How long have you been planning this?"

"I have been thinking about it for awhile now, but it all came together in the middle of the night, last Sunday. I went to the jewelers on Monday and made the arrangements with the restaurant. Of course, I had no idea what I would be facing for the rest of the week, but everything came together in the end."

"Do you mean you already had this planned when you took me bowling Monday night?"

"Yes, and I almost went crazy trying to keep it a secret."

Most of the people in the restaurant had left, but the waiter came over and told them to take their time. They were eager to discuss their future plans.

"Do you know if your nursing graduation will be separate from the college grad?"

"I really don't know, but I can probably ask one of the instructors and find out."

"I understand the regular graduation is the first Saturday in June, so we could easily have our wedding around the middle of June. What do you think?"

"That sounds good Allen; how do you feel about a big wedding?"

"I don't know. I think I prefer something small, family only maybe?"

"Well, I promised my classmates they would all be invited. I have always dreamed about having a big wedding."

"So much money is wasted on a big wedding, I'd rather have that money to put a down payment on our first home."

"But think of the memories we would treasure for the rest of our lives."

"Maybe we should talk this over with my parents tomorrow, and yours after that, okay?"

"Sounds good. They can make some suggestions; my folks would pay for most of it, you know."

"Whatever, Pumpkin."

"It would be best to see my folks next weekend before semester break ends on Monday, okay?"

"Sounds good to me."

They realized Jan had to get back to the dorm, so Allen took care of the bill. The waiter had wrapped Jan's dinner in foil and presented it to her in the shape of a dove. Before Allen opened the car door for Jan, he took her into his arms and kissed her the way he had last Sunday-not once, not twice, but three times. They talked all the way home, and as he walked her to the door, even though he knew that curious eyes were watching, he kissed her again.

Jan walked inside, and everyone started jumping up and down, all asking questions at once. Jan decided not to say a word. She just raised her left hand and wiggled her fingers. Hysteria rained at the nurses' dormitory!

* * *

Allen called Jan Sunday morning greeting her with, "How's my beautiful fiancé this morning?"

"Still in a state of euphoria, and my feet haven't touched the ground yet!"

"Not to worry. They say that wears off after you've been married for fifty years."

"So, that's what I have to look forward to?"

"Indeed, you do, my darling. Just got off the phone with mom, and she told me the ambulance should be arriving at the med center between one and two this afternoon. So, I was wondering if you might be interested in having lunch out with your future husband, followed by some time together waiting for the folks to arrive?"

Jan's stomach did a flip flop when he said the word husband. She took a deep breath to compose herself before answering, "Sounds absolutely smashing."

"I'll pick you up in 30 minutes, my sweet lady."

"See you then."

Jan started looking through her closet again to decide what to wear. She settled on some white tailored slacks with a red blouse trimmed in white and her white pumps. Mandy volunteered to work on her hair again and help Jan with her make-up. Jan hugged Mandy to thank her and went downstairs to wait. They met half way up the walk. He hugged her and kissed her, and neither of them cared anymore who might be watching.

He took her to an ice cream shop, for a hot dog and a root beer float. Allen said, "You know I have more schooling after you pass your state boards, and then I'll intern with an established dentist."

"Yes, I realize that, and I want to work until we start a family. I also would like to continue college and work towards my masters degree. Actually, I would like to be instrumental in bringing about some changes in many antiquated policies here at the med center."

"I guess I just want to make it clear, you will be the primary bread winner for awhile. Are you okay with that?"

"You know, I hadn't even thought about it in those terms; I'm fine with us working as a team to achieve our goals. Whatever it takes."

"That's what I love about you. You're willing to walk the path no matter how many mud slides you encounter."

"As long as we are together, I'll go through a few floods as well. Oh, by the way, I'm going to see Carol tomorrow night, and I just have a feeling she has some good news about the witch."

"Good. Did Carol throw cold water on her and watch her melt?"

"I wouldn't put it past her."

"You know, I'd like to meet this Carol. I have next Thursday off. Do you think she would be free?"

"Funny you asked. She wants to meet you too. I'll ask her on Monday."

CHAPTER TWENTY TWO
THE BOMB TO THE DOC'S LIBIDO

When Allen and Jan arrived at the hospital, Jan inquired what room Frank Morris would be in. They decided to go up and wait there. They found the room empty, each sitting down in a chair and discussed where they should get married. They both agreed they had a lot of friends from college and the hospital, and maybe it would be best to be married in town. Then Jan brought up that they each had a lot of family and friends in their own home towns, many who would not be able to travel far. They looked at each other and Allen said, "How do we work that out?"

They agreed they should talk it over with both sets of parents and decide from there.

During a lull in the conversation, Allen got up from his chair, closed the door to the room and brought Jan to a standing position. He took advantage of this opportunity to wrap her in his arms and kiss her with the passion of two people very much in love. Just as he stopped and was looking into her eyes, the door opened. They both jumped, and a sweet voice said, "Oh I'm so sorry, I was . . . is that you Allen?"

He turned around, grinning sheepishly. "Oh hello Aunt Barbara."

"Is it alright if I come in?"

"Yes, of course, and I would like you to meet my fiancé, Janet Watkins, I mean Winston."

"Well, I'm very glad to meet you, Janet," reaching to give her a quick hug. "Your mother didn't mention that you were engaged, Allen."

"She doesn't know about it yet. I just asked Jan to marry me last night. I plan to break the news to both of them today."

"Oh, my goodness. I promise I won't say a word when they get here. They should be coming in any minute; I saw Frank arrive in the ambulance just before I came up here."

Allen got another chair for his aunt and found another across the hall for his mom. Just then his mom arrived and gave hugs to everyone saying, "Your dad is on his way up now."

Jan felt a tingle of excitement while awaiting his arrival after Allen had described the positive changes that his dad had made. At one time she wasn't sure she ever wanted to see him again.

They heard some commotion down the hall coupled with laughter. Allen laughed out loud and said, "My dad has arrived."

Barbara chimed in, "Sounds like I have my brother back."

Carmela grinned, "Yes, he most definitely is back."

Jan could hardly wait to see him.

*　*　*

They could not stop laughing; Allen's father was keeping everyone in stitches. The ambulance drivers had just settled him in bed when he took hold of one of their arms and said, "Hey fellas, before you leave I think you should fill a couple of syringes with the same stuff you gave me for the trip and pass them around so we all can feel this good!"

They laughed, patting his arm, and said, "We really enjoyed getting to know you Frank. You kept us entertained all the way down. Good luck, sir. We hope to see you again."

"Thanks, guys. You're good young men."

Frank looked around the room and pointed his left hand toward Barbara and said, "Hey sis, come over here and give your big brother a kiss." She walked over and kissed him, and then he patted her arm. "I want to thank you, sweetheart, for letting Carmela stay with you while I'm down here."

She kissed him again saying, "It's really my pleasure. My house is very lonely since Bert died and I look forward to having company."

Carmela moved up beside Barbara, and put an arm around her. "You know, Frank, Barb and I have always been more like sisters than in-laws."

Allen took Jan's hand, and together they walked over to the other side of the bed so they could see both of his parents' faces. He cleared his throat and said, "Mom and Dad, Jan and I have something to tell you. Last night I took Jan to a restaurant and asked her to marry me when we graduate."

Jan held up her left hand she had been discreetly hiding until now. All three started asking questions at once while Allen's mom gave them both a hug, followed by Aunt Barbara.

Allen's dad said, "Hold that hand up where I can really see it, Janet. Wow, Allen, did you rob a bank to buy that?" He gave Allen a wink and a smile.

Mom spoke up. "Let's all go over and sit down so you can tell us all about last night and what your future plans are."

Allen and Jan took turns revealing the details of their night out and the excitement of everyone in the restaurant. "Jan and I agree, we want to finish this year of college before we marry."

Jan spoke up, "We do have one problem and we need your opinion on where we might have our wedding because we have friends and family that live in our respective home towns."

Allen's dad was the first to speak. "If you ask me, and I think you did, you plan a big wedding here and send out your invites early to everyone, and if they can't come that's okay. They'll get plenty of chances to meet the newlyweds later. What do you think mom?"

Allen interrupted, "I really don't want a big wedding. Let's keep it to family and our closest friends."

"Allen, I told you last night, I've always had my heart set on a big wedding."

"Pumpkin, we can save so much money if we have a small wedding, and it will be just as binding as a big one."

Jan was feeling angry, and she wasn't sure why as she blurted out, "So you don't care how I feel about it!"

"Jan, I'm just trying to be practical!" Allen's voice escalated.

Dad intervened. "Jan, may I ask you a question?"

Oh, no. He's going to side with Allen. "Yes, I guess so."

"Can your parent's afford the expense of a big wedding?"

"Yes, of course they can."

"Allen, let me tell you something I have learned over the years. Women are ruled by their heart, and men are ruled by their intellect. As men, we need to listen to what is in a woman's heart and learn compassion from them. Woman need to listen to a man's ability to analyze. What I'm saying, son, is let your sweetheart have a big wedding, and she will make you grateful for the rest of your life; if you don't, she'll make your life miserable!"

Everyone laughed, and the situation was de-clawed.

Allen walked over, kneeling down in front of Jan and said, "First of all, can you forgive me for not listening to your heart?"

"Are you saying we can have a big wedding?"

"Yes, absolutely."

"Okay, I forgive you," she said as she threw her arms around him and kissed him.

Allen's mom had been deep in thought through all of this; she lifted her head and said, "I think your dad is right, and I also think I can arrange a bridal shower at our house a couple of months before the wedding and invite local friends. Then if they can't travel to the wedding, they shouldn't feel so bad. What do you kids think?"

Jan answered, "I think that would be wonderful. Thanks mom."

Aunt Barbara spoke up, saying, "I would like to offer my home to anyone in the family who needs a place to stay for the wedding, including your parents, Jan."

"I think they will probably stay with their cousins, Carol Lee and Otto, but thank you for offering."

Jan looked at Allen's dad and changed the subject. "Frank, are you alright? You look a bit tired."

"No, I was just realizing I could easily become a grandpa before I turn sixty."

Allen and Jan laughed, as Allen replied, "Hey, dad, we aren't even married yet. Don't push it."

Frank got very quiet and with some hesitancy said, "I can't believe that I'm actually alive and able to be a part of my son's joy." He looked right at Jan. "I hope that you will find I am a much different person than the one you met a little over a year ago. That horrible man died at the bottom of a mine shaft, and I pray that you can forgive me for treating you so badly, Janet. I can tell you are the best thing that has ever happened to my son, and I'm thrilled to accept you as a part of our family." He smiled a bit, still gazing at Jan. "Would you humor an old dilapidated man and call me dad? But only if you feel comfortable."

Jan got up, walked over to his side, leaned down and kissed his cheek. "I would considerate it an honor, dad. And thank you for giving your wonderful son some fatherly advice. Are you sure you're the same person I met last year?"

Frank became tearful. "I'm definitely not that guy and never will be again. Hey, we need to stop this serious stuff. Nurse Jan, did you notice that I can use my left arm more? The nurses and physical therapist have been working on it. Course, this sling won't let me move the right; since I'm going to have surgery tomorrow, will you be able to stop by afterward?"

"Yes, Dad, I intend to keep a close eye on you while you're here, okay?"

He peeked his head around Jan and with a big smile said to the others, "We are going to have an honest to goodness real nurse in the family, and on top of that, I'm finally going to have a daughter!"

Everyone laughed while Jan walked over and sat down.

Allen looked at the three women and said, "Would you ladies mind going for a little walk or something? I would like to have a private talk with my father."

They willingly left to get a drink and some exercise while Allen closed the door and turned to his dad asking, "Dad, do you mind if we talk about the box?"

His dad snickered, answering, "Not at all. Tell me, how long did it take for you to get over the shock?"

"Dad, I'm still in a state of shock, and I really appreciate what you did for me, but why did you give me cash?"

"Well son, you have to realize I knew these guys were determined to do me in, and I was pretty sure that I would be dead within a few hours or days. I thought about writing a check, but what if your bank wouldn't honor such a large sum of money? Besides, I kind of enjoyed the thought of you opening it and receiving the shock of your life. Have you told anyone about it?

"Absolutely not. Have you?"

"Son, there are no secrets between your mom and I. She now knows all about it."

"Well, since Jan is my future wife, can I tell her now?"

"I really don't think that would be wise. Besides I specified your *wife*. Future was not mentioned, right?"

"Okay, I get your point. Dad, you've no idea what this means to me, especially the words in your letter and the promise that I have my real father back in my life." He took his left hand and said, "Thank you. I love you so much."

"I love you too. Hope you didn't mind me speaking about your wedding."

"No, Dad; I think I really needed to hear your advice. I could tell Jan was ready to blow her pressure gauge."

"Okay, now go find those beautiful ladies and bring them back to brighten up this room. And by the way, son, I really love the one with that big rock on her hand."

"You know what, Dad? I do too."

He found the girls walking down the hall, Jan was animated in her conversation to them.

She started towards Allen when she saw Mrs. Novak coming down the hall. Her instructor walked up to her giving her a hug exclaiming, "I haven't seen you forever, Miss Winston. How are you?"

"I couldn't be better." Then Jan turned to introduce Mrs. Novak to everyone, and when she mentioned the word fiancé" Mrs. Novak had to hug her again.

Mrs. Novak said, "Well congratulations. And I have a surprise for you. I've been promoted."

"That's great. What have you been promoted to?"

"An instructor in the nursing program."

Jan jumped up and down saying, "That's wonderful. You will be a great teacher, and I hope you will be able to work with me during my senior year. I'm so excited for you."

"I am too. Nice meeting everyone. I have to run, but I'll see you soon, Miss Winston."

They entered the room just as the nurse had finished giving Frank a shot for pain. "He's probably going to get sleepy now, so when he drifts off, it will give you all an opportunity to get some dinner."

Just as she left, Dr. Worthington walked in. He looked at Frank and introduced himself as his surgeon, turning as he said, "And this must be your family." He paused for a second and asked, "Miss Winston, is that you?"

His eyes took her in from top to bottom.

"Yes, and this is my fiancé, Allen Morris, his mother Carmela Morris and his aunt, Barbara."

Jan wanted to laugh at the look on his face when she said fiancé.

He politely shook hands then turned back to Frank, saying, "I will be your surgeon tomorrow, with another doctor assisting me. Frank, I want you to know that this will be a very complicated surgery. From what I can determine, after looking at the x-rays, I will have some major repair work to do." He turned to Carmela and continued, "You can expect him to be in surgery around four hours, and I will likely keep him in recovery room longer than usual to monitor him closely." He turned back to Frank. "We will be sending you up to the orthopedic floor after a few days to start your physical therapy. Your recovery and ability to use that arm again, will be determined by your capability to push yourself through excruciating pain. That is, if you want to regain full range of motion. Any questions?"

Frank looked at him with a sense of determination on his face and said, "You fix it doc, and I'll work it, okay?"

Dr. Worthington gave him a smile, then turned toward Jan and said, "Engaged? What a shame! But congratulations to you both." He turned on his heel and left.

Jan giggled as soon as he closed the door behind him and told the family he was somewhat of a playboy but definitely the best surgeon in the state.

Frank was sleepy, so they went to the cafeteria. She saw some of her fellow students there and went over to tell them about Mrs. Novak. They were all excited because everybody liked her. She was always so fair and helpful to the students.

One of the girls asked Jan, "Does anyone know where Mrs. Stewart is? She hasn't been seen anywhere in the last week or so."

"I don't know yet, but I have a feeling I'll find out from Carol tomorrow night. She told me yesterday she had some news with a great big grin on her face. Maybe she's gone. Let's not get our hopes up. It may be too good to be true."

She turned and went to sit down with Allen. Mom sat quietly looking at her plate and said, "I'm really worried about Frank's surgery tomorrow after what the doctor said."

Jan put her hand over hers. "Mom, I'm confident everything's going to be alright. If dad could live through being thrown down a mineshaft and lay there in agony for four days without food or water, I think he's strong enough to get through this surgery."

"I hadn't thought about it that way, honey. I'm sure you're right. He has a very strong will, and especially now that he has come to his senses and wants to re-establish his relationship with his family."

Barbara leaned forward, "Don't forget he wants to be around for those grandchildren."

Jan felt her cheeks get hot as she glanced at Allen, then she put her eyes down.

Aunt Barbara was staring at Allen when she blurted out, "Allen, when did you pick up the obnoxious habit of chewing gum all the time?"

Allen's mouth dropped open as he shockingly said, "I didn't know it was obnoxious!"

"Well, I'm sorry, but it is, and I apologize for mouthing off about it."

Allen looked around at his mother and Jan. "Does anyone else agree with Aunt Barb?"

Jan put her head down and slowly lifted her right hand. Then out of the corner of her eye she saw his mom do the same.

Allen shook his head and said, "Well thanks for letting me know! Why hasn't anyone mentioned this before?"

Jan quietly said, "I didn't want to offend you and it certainly was a better habit than smoking."

Mom snickered. "I've been meaning to tell you for a long time, but I figured you had enough on your plate with your father and then a girlfriend and college, and I just tried to overlook it."

Allen grabbed a paper napkin, took the gum from his mouth, took a pack out of his pocket and threw them all in the garbage can. "I wish to make just one request. Please tell me up front if I have a bad habit, okay?"

Everyone said, "Okay."

Jan changed the subject as she started talking about her rotation tomorrow.

CHAPTER TWENTY THREE

A MIRACLE

Jan bypassed the elevator, and ran up the stairs to the third floor, her heart pounding with every step in anticipation of her next assignment. She felt absolutely giddy as she approached the double doors that said "AUTHORIZED PERSONNEL ONLY." Pushing them open, she approached the nurses' station.

Mrs. Novak sat smiling at her, with her hands folded on the desk. Jan walked up smiling expectantly and asked, "Are you my instructor in labor and delivery?"

"I am, Miss Winston, and we'll learn together since this is my first day also."

Just then a very young nurse walked in, introduced herself as Miss Burton, the Day Supervisor for Labor and Delivery. Radiating a lovely smile, she said, "I'm here to show you around, and since you are both new, you can do a lot of observing today."

Jan loved nurses like her and hoped she could develop the same kind of qualities in her career. She judged her to be in her early twenties (maybe close to Jan's age). She had chocolate brown skin, sparkling black eyes and tightly curled hair, cut very short. She was a couple of inches taller than Jan and stunningly beautiful. *She could be a model or a movie star.*

Miss Burton walked them down the hall to where there were a few mothers in different stages of labor. Most of them had their husbands with them, and one looked quite young with only her mother in attendance. Miss Burton walked into each room, introducing Jan and Mrs. Novak.

They went back down the hall and through another set of double doors labeled with the warning sign "NO ADMITTANCE" on it. The nurse supervisor then escorted them into a room and said, "This is one of our delivery rooms. We have four, all primarily the same with one set up for multiple birth deliveries." She explained the different types of equipment and then turned to leave.

Jan took this opportunity to ask a question she'd been stifling. "Miss Burton, is there any chance we will actually see a delivery today?"

The nurse smiled and answered, "Most definitely. We have a couple of mothers getting pretty close, and we don't want you to miss out on such a privilege."

Jan beamed and said, "Oh, I can't wait!"

Mrs. Novak laughed and said, "After having two of my own, I don't have the same enthusiasm Miss Winston has."

They continued through another door and could hear the distinctive cries of newborns. Miss Burton introduced them to the nursery. They followed her in. She turned at the door. "We put on a gown and mask before entering the nursery." Jan recalled the time Miss Kingston had brought the class to this area to see a sadly deformed newborn.

Miss Burton picked up one of the crying babies, gently giving it some pats on its back until it gave out a loud belch. She cuddled it a bit and then went to return it to another bassinet.

Jan asked, "Why are you putting him in another bassinet?"

"Miss Winston, you get the gold star for that question. That was kind of a dirty trick, but I wanted to see if you were observing. Our rule is, when you have held any baby, you always check the baby's bracelet with the mom's name on the crib before returning it to its designated bassinet. Then she beckoned them to follow her into a doorway at the back of the room as she said, "I'll now show you the premature nursery."

Three tiny babies in incubators looked more like little dolls than real babies. Each infant had a tiny tube going into their nose to their stomachs for nourishment. Jan had never seen such small little needles inserted in the side of their temples with an IV attached. An RN was there, and she asked Jan to sit in a chair. She opened an incubator, picked up one of the babies and placed it in Jan's arms. Jan was in awe of this tiny human being as she looked at the delicate little infant in her arms who looked more like a doll than a baby. She was afraid if she moved even an inch this delicate angel would break. Jan was grateful the baby was sleeping as Miss Burton pointed out many pieces of equipment that Jan had never seen before, all of them geared to the size of these tiny babies. The nurse then took the baby from her which startled the infant, and its delicate arms made an arch like movement as the nurse placed it back in the incubator. Jan asked if the mothers were allowed to hold their babies, and Miss Burton answered, "Oh, no. It's against the rules, but they can look through that window over there and we will hold up their infant so they can see them." Once again, Jan felt the urge to say, *That's not right. If I can be in here, why not the mother who gave them birth?*

They left the nursery, and went out the double doors to another hall called "Postpartum." This was like the rest of the hospital-just a place for mothers to heal from their delivery. Miss Burton explained that the nurses taught the mothers how to nurse or feed their babies, and the infants were brought to them on a regular basis for feedings. Mothers and babies were sent home, as long as both were doing well, on the third or fourth day after delivery, or five to seven days following a C-section.

Miss Burton spoke directly to Jan. "You will be rotated through each area that you have seen, as assigned by Mrs. Novak. Do you have any questions?"

"Not at the moment."

"Okay, I suggest that you read the charts of the mothers in labor, take an early lunch break, then come back to follow one of our mothers to the delivery room."

Miss Burton showed them the chart rack, and they each took a chart, sat down at the desk and began reading. Jan realized she had picked up the chart of the young mother as she began to read. The chart lacked a last name, identifying her only as Melinda. Apparently she had spent most of her pregnancy at a nearby home for unwed mothers away from the city where she lived. Her mother was here to help her through labor, then the baby would be adopted by a couple that had been screened and interviewed, eagerly awaiting the birth if their baby.

Jan tried to visualize what it must be like to carry a baby for nine months, feeling the life within, and then giving it away. The mother had just turned seventeen, which would mean the baby was conceived when she was sixteen.

She turned to Mrs. Novak. "Could I discuss this patient with you? I'd like to know more about this home for unwed mothers; I've never heard of this before."

"Sure. These homes were originally developed through the Catholic Church and staffed with nuns. Now there are some privately owned homes. The girls are given a small room, usually shared with a roommate. They have their own bed and dresser. They eat together in a common dining area; they're assigned certain chores to do and given classes to keep up with their school work. Counseling is made available, but they are given the choice to keep the child or have it adopted. Adoption is highly encouraged almost to the point of being mandatory. But the final decision is theirs. The girls know nothing about the adopting parents and sign documents to release all parental rights."

"What a sad predicament to be in at such a young age."

"I agree. Parents and teachers need to be more open about teenage pregnancy. It's such a hush-hush subject."

"You're right. We need to break that mold."

They continued to study the rest of the charts, including some that were in surgery having a C- section. Mrs. Novak told Jan she would be able to follow mothers through to surgery when they had to have their babies by cesarean. Jan looked forward to it.

Jan looked at Mrs. Novak and asked, "Can you go to lunch with me?"

Mrs. Novak smiled and said, "I don't see why not, since we are bound together with adhesive tape for the day. Let's go."

As they were eating lunch, Mrs. Novak asked, "Where's your engagement ring?"

"Oh, I pinned it with a safety pin to the inside of my pocket, so it's always close to me." She pulled open the pocket on her apron, unpinned it and handed it to Mrs. Novak. Jan, let out a deep sigh. "I wish I could wear it all of the time, but it's so against the stupid rules."

"I know honey, it doesn't make a lot of sense since we married nurses are allowed to wear them unless we're in surgery." She looked at the ring up close. Wow this is beautiful! He spent a lot of money on you. That is one huge diamond. I would say you have found a man that is head over heels in love with you. Congratulations."

"Thanks. The feeling is mutual; I wish we didn't have to wait until graduation."

"Is that still the rule?"

"Yes, but it was always my choice also. I just don't want to mix school and studies with a new marriage."

"You're right. Good thinking. But you only have about, what, eleven months to wait, right?"

"Yes, but it's getting harder to wait every time I'm with him."

"Honey, I was a virgin when my husband and I got married, and I can honestly tell you, it was so well worth the wait and still is, believe me."

"Thanks, Mrs. Novak, I needed to hear that."

"Hey, pin this in your pocket, and we better get back. Don't want you to miss out on the fun, right?"

"Let's go."

As they went through the double doors, they could hear some loud moaning and wondered if they'd missed something. Miss Burton came out of one of the rooms. Walking toward them, she said, "Why don't you both go into that room and just observe. She's about nine centimeters dilated, and her contractions are two minutes apart. The mother's name is Maria Olivera. She and her husband are expecting you."

They walked in and thanked the Oliveras for letting them observe, and then politely stood out of the way and watched. Jan could tell Maria was getting very little rest between contractions. She was perspiring heavily and moaning loudly with each one. Her husband had a damp washcloth that he kept to wipe her brow. He gave her some ice chips to soothe her.

He turned toward them. "I feel like I should be doing something more to help her. Do you have any suggestions?"

Mrs. Novak stepped over to the bed. "You can try massaging her back; here let me show you how."

"Does that feel good, Maria?"

"Yes, please keep doing it." Her husband took over, as Mrs. Novak coached him.

"Is this your first baby, Ruben?"

"Yes, it is. We are very excited but a little bit scared too."

"Do you have anyone to help you when you take her home?"

"Oh, yes, plenty of family, maybe a little too much even."

"Well, that's good. Better too much than too little."

Mrs. Novak came back over by Jan.

Just then Maria had a contraction that made her scream, "Please give me something to stop the pain!"

Jan thought *There must be something they could do for her!* She whispered in Mrs. Novak's ear, "Isn't there something they can give her?"

"They can't give her anything now, but when she gets into delivery, the doctor will offer the option of an epidural-an injection into the spine to anesthetize from the waist down."

Jan watched as Maria's contractions escalated non-stop, and listened to her screams getting louder. Miss Burton came in to check her and began moving full speed ahead.

"Mr. Olivera, we are going to move your wife to the delivery room. Mrs. Novak will show you to the father's waiting room. Miss Winston, help me transfer Maria to a gurney and come with me."

In the delivery room, they transferred Maria to the delivery table, put her feet in the stirrups and put some kind of antiseptic solution on her legs and birthing area. Jan noticed Maria's entire birthing area had been shaved earlier and it looked like she was bulging outward. The doctor entered, put on his gown and gloves and asked Maria if she had changed her mind about wanting an epidural. She said no, and he proceeded with his examination. Then he left the room saying, "Call me when she's ready." *How odd, why doesn't he stay to coach her through this part?* They gave her some oxygen with a mask, and Jan stood back to watch.

Mrs. Novak came in, joining Jan. She could see a circle of black in the birth canal and asked Mrs. Novak what that was. When she told Jan it's the hair on the baby's head, Jan wanted to whoop and holler with excitement. The nurses coached Maria to push during each contraction.

After a few minutes the doctor reappeared, took his place on a stool and did a quick episiotomy, which is an incision made at the birth canal to widen it. Maria pushed a couple of more times and the head emerged. The doctor maneuvered the baby around a bit, helping one shoulder and the next, as the baby slid out into the doctor's waiting hands.

"Maria, congratulations --- you have a beautiful baby girl." he told her. After suctioning and cutting the umbilical cord, the doctor stood her up and laid her on Maria's chest. Emotion swept through the room as we shed some tears with Maria.

What a miracle, to witness the joy of a live birth on Jan's first day in labor and delivery. She watched as the nurses cleaned the baby, put drops in her eyes, and took footprints of her feet. They placed a tiny bracelet made from little alphabet beads spelling Maria's name on the baby. Then they wrapped her in a pink receiving blanket and let mommy hold her for another minute before taking the baby to the nursery.

In the meantime, Jan observed the doctor stitch Maria's episiotomy. Then she stood in awe as she watched the delivery of the placenta.

She whispered to Mrs. Novak, "It's amazing how two cells come together, then nine months later a full-sized infant comes out to greet the world. It's a real miracle."

The doctor stripped off his gown and gloves, and leaned down to Maria saying, "You did really good, honey. Now I'll go out and tell your husband the good news."

Jan turned to her instructor and asked, "Why isn't the father in here during delivery?"

"It's against hospital rules. I think they're afraid they might get sick or faint."

"Hmm, that's interesting." Jan thought *I want my husband with me when I give birth.*

Jan had just enough time to see Maria in a wheel chair and her husband looking through the nursery window at their new baby girl. They were both crying tears of joy.

CHAPTER TWENTY FOUR
"HO, HO, THE WITCH IS DEAD"

As soon as Jan left the third floor, she went to the room of her future father-in-law. She found Allen and his mom there. Frank was still in recovery. Allen stood up and kissed Jan lightly on the cheek then offered her his chair. She turned and hugged his mom, then asked, "Any news?"

Allen answered, "The surgery took a little over five hours, and the doc said it was like a jigsaw puzzle inside his shoulder. Dad held up real good during the surgery, but he's had a hard time coming out of the anesthesia, even though the doctor says it's nothing to worry about."

"When do you think he'll get back to his room?"

Mom answered, "Any time now, I hope."

Allen said, "I sure hope so because I promised my boss I would be at the station in forty five minutes. Hey, beautiful, you do look extra cute in your nurses uniform."

Jan giggled and said, "Yeah, I can hardly wait to get into something more comfortable. You will never believe what I saw today."

"Okay, Pumpkin, what won't I believe you saw today?"

"I actually saw a mother give birth to a beautiful baby girl. It was the most exciting thing I've ever witnessed."

"More exciting than watching me chew gum?"

"Oh Allen, are you never going to let me live that one down?"

"Do you remember the three things you made me commit to when we first decided to date each other exclusively?"

"I know, I know! To always be honest with each other. I goofed, okay? So I apologize, now can we go on with the rest of our lives?"

"You're so cute when you get irritated."

"Allen, enough!"

"Alright already. You know I love you."

"And I love you too."

Allen's Mom spoke up. "Seeing a baby born --- that's wonderful, Jan. I wish I could have seen my baby boy born, but they had to put me out because he was being born backwards or sideways or something like that, and the doctor had to reach inside of me and turn the baby around. They said he was born blue, and they didn't expect him to live. They told me I was so badly damaged, they did an emergency hysterectomy or I wouldn't have survived." Carmela wrapped her arms around Allen, "I didn't even know I had a son until 24 hours after he was born!"

Jan hugged them both, "Well, I'm sure glad you both survived because I don't think I want to marry anyone else but him."

They heard voices approaching, and Doctor Worthington came through the door followed by the nurses and an orderly wheeling Frank in on a gurney. The doctor walked over to Carmela and said "He finally came around; seems to be doing fine now. We will keep him heavily sedated for a couple of days, or he would be in a whole world of hurt!" He glanced at Jan, then over to Allen and said, "You sure are a lucky guy." Out the door he went.

Mom went over beside Frank's bed, looked at the massive bandage around her husband's right arm and shoulder, then shook her head as she started to cry. Allen and Jan put their arms protectively around her and let her sob in their arms.

Completely oblivious to anything other than the drug induced circles of fantasy decorating his mind, Frank snored away.

Allen released his arms and said, "I hate to break this up, but I really have to go to work."

Turning to Jan he said, "May I escort you to your quarters, madam?"

She gave a little curtsy and answered, "Only if you promise to marry me in eleven months, sir."

"Mmm, I will have to give that some serious thought because I'm already spoken for."

Mom interrupted, saying, "Oh, go on you two, and I'll see you tomorrow."

Allen led Jan to the elevator hoping that they could be alone as they went downstairs, but several people came along with them. As they were about to step off, he held Jan back, closed the door and pushed the up button. He gently pushed her against the wall and kissed her until the elevator came to a stop. As others came aboard, they stood close together holding hands, smiling like the fish that got away after grabbing the bait.

The last thing they wanted to do was separate, but he had to go to work, and she was going to see Carol, so he pecked her on the cheek, went to his car and she went to the dorm to change her clothes.

* * *

Carol greeted her with a hug, "Come in for some cookies and milk." They sat together at her little table in the kitchen.

"Carol, I'm so excited, I saw an actual delivery of a baby today."

"Well, you're one up on me, I've never had one or seen one. That must have been a thrill, are mommy and baby doing okay?"

"Oh, they're fine. How are all the children?

"Nothing much has changed, we have some new students, but you already knew that."

"Carol, what's your big news?"

"It finally happened! The RNs plus two of the caretakers, one of them myself, paid a visit to Mrs. Caspar, the Director of Nursing Services, who is ultimately Miss Kingston's boss. We came up with this idea at a strategy meeting prior to the visit. Since Mrs. Stewart and Miss Kingston are sisters, we didn't feel right about approaching Miss Kingston. We explained to Mrs. Caspar the actions and behavior of Mrs. Stewart towards the student nurses, the staff and the children. She asked for specific details of her behavior, and we replayed the scenes we had each personally witnessed. She was mortified to say the least!"

"What happened next?"

"While we were still there, she called to see if Miss Kingston could come to her office. You should have seen the look on Miss K's face when she walked in."

"Did she say anything?"

"Nope, she just sat down and looked straight at Mrs. Caspar."

"We had to repeat everything for Miss Kingston's benefit. She put her head down and just shook it back and forth. When we finished, she said, "I'm so very sorry, and I take full responsibility for Mrs. Stewart and apologize for the damage she's done. I'm truly sorry for her behavior and I will take action immediately."

Carol added, "Then, Mrs. Caspar excused us and later we heard Mrs. Stewart's nursing license was revoked and Miss K. sent her to live with their cousin in New York to procure employment in some other field.

"Wow. How did you feel when you left the director's office?" Jan asked.

"Well, we were relieved that Mrs. Caspar listened to us and she made us feel justified in talking to her."

"That's great. Carol, now I have some news."

"What's that, Jan?"

"Have you ever worked with Mrs. Novak?"

"No, honey, I don't even know what she looks like. Why do you ask?"

"She was the RN on the medical floor my first day in the hospital. She was so nice to me. I could hardly believe it. And now she has taken Mrs. Stewart's place as an instructor in labor and delivery and the Children's Home. You will really like her. I'm sure of that."

Carol said, "Whew. What a relief."

"Now Carol, I have some really exciting news." She raised her left hand as she continued. "I'm engaged to be married next June!"

Carol looked at her ring and gave her a big hug. "I'm so happy for you."

"I can bring Allen over Thursday to meet you, if that works for you?"

"Okay. Why don't I have the two of you over for dinner. We can visit for a little while until you have to get back to hitting the books. How does that sound?"

"That sounds exciting, Carol. You are such a wonderful friend, and I'm so grateful you took the initiative to rally the troops and visit Mrs. Caspar."

"You know, I really feel sorry for Miss Kingston. She was just trying to help a sister that never should have gone into this profession in the first place, but she realizes now that it was the wrong thing to do. Her sister moved out the next day, and the last I heard she's doing well with her cousin who's getting her a job in an assembly plant. Miss Kingston told me she has been in and out of mental institutions all of her life. Isn't that sad?"

"It is! But I don't feel bad at all now that she is far away from our precious children. Did you know that Kim would like to work there when she graduates? Didn't she do wonders with Katrina?"

"Yes, and Kim will be coming on Sundays to spend a couple of hours singing and dancing with her. What a sweetheart."

"Carol, I really have to go. That alarm goes off very early in the morning. I hate getting up in the dark. I love you, Carol, and we'll see you Thursday. Okay?"

You bet, honey. Can't wait to meet your Mr. Twinkle Toes."

Jan laughed as she gave her a hug and went out the door.

Jan took a quick detour through the hospital to look in on Frank. She found him alone and barely awake, she gave him a kiss on his cheek and whispered, "I'll come by tomorrow. He was awake just enough to wink and say, "I love you, Jan."

Her response surprised even her as she said, "I love you, too."

CHAPTER TWENTY FIVE
A SURPRISE PACKAGE

The next morning she eagerly went to her assignment, anticipating another exciting day. She was assigned to postpartum and one of her patients was Maria. Jan got Maria up to walk down the hall for a minute, and then she sat in a chair while Jan made her bed.

Maria looked at Jan and asked, "Have you ever had a baby?"

Jan answered, "No, I'm not married yet. We're waiting until I graduate next June, and then I hope I don't get pregnant right away. I would like to wait at least a couple of years."

Maria started to laugh as she said, "That's what we said and look, ten months later we have a baby!"

"I know, you can't always plan these things ahead. You never know what might happen. How do you feel about labor now that it's over?"

She giggled again and answered, "Right now I don't think I ever want to go through that again."

"I can understand. You had a pretty rough time of it that last hour or so. But you refused the doctor's offer to give you an epidural. That would have given you some relief in the delivery room. Can you tell me why you declined it?"

"Oh, Miss Winston, I have a younger brother who is paralyzed from the waist down due to a motorcycle accident, and I didn't want to experience that even for a few hours. Also, I have heard that it can result in a permanent paralysis if the doctor makes a slight mistake. No way, it just wasn't for me."

"Well, I can certainly understand that, but I really don't think that it happens very often from the doctor making a mistake."

"Who made a mistake?" Mrs. Novak asked as she came through the door.

"Oh good," Jan turned towards her. Maybe you can clarify our question. Maria, tell Mrs. Novak why you didn't have the epidural."

While Maria explained, Jan completed the bed and waited for Mrs. Novak to answer. After listening intently, her instructor said, "Well, I understand your fear, but the fact is that permanent paralysis resulting from an epidural is about a million to one. It is actually a relatively easy procedure for the doctor and very difficult to make a mistake. I have never hesitated to have it done and it is such a tremendous relief."

Maria looked at Jan and then at Mrs. Novak. "I guess my fear was unreasonable. I'll consider it next time around."

Jan helped Maria back to bed just as her baby was brought in. The RN stayed with Maria to help her with breast feeding. The nurse explained, "The fluid she receives in these first feedings is called colostrums. It's like giving your baby a booster shot of immunity." Jan showed Maria how to hold her baby while feeding and ways to burp her. When she finished, Jan went in to her next patient.

When Jan entered Melinda's room, she found her curled in a fetal position, quietly sobbing. Her heart went out to her as she walked over to the bed and started rubbing her back. "Melinda, I'm sorry you've had to go through this; I'm sure it's very hard on you."

Melinda turned to Jan and said, "I'm such an awful person. I wish I were dead!"

"I know you feel this way right now, but I want you to know that you're my hero for not having an abortion. By giving a wonderful couple the gift of your baby, his parents will be filled with love and appreciation for you."

Melinda turned towards Jan, as she wiped the tears from her cheeks with the palms of her hands, and softly whimpered, "I never thought of it that way. My boyfriend was a lot older than me, and when I told him I was pregnant, he called me terrible names. "I'll have nothing to do with your baby! Then he left town. I should have listened to my mother. She kept telling me he was too old and stringing me along. In the beginning, he told me he loved me; when I was scared that I might get pregnant, he told me everything would be okay. He said he loved me and wanted to marry me when I turned eighteen. Oh, I was such a fool to believe him!"

"Melinda, you're not a bad person. You were just very gullible and fell for one of the oldest lines in the world. Now you've had to grow up very fast, but you can go back to school and keep your head up high because you have done the right thing. Don't you ever be ashamed of what you've done, even if you kept your baby and struggled through raising it yourself, you should not feel ashamed. Yes, you made a mistake, but you've made it right in the end."

Jan helped her get up, and together they took a walk down the hall. As they came back to her room, they heard a baby cry, and Melinda hesitated as she asked Jan, "Do you think my baby is crying a lot?"

"Most babies cry a lot when they are newborns."

"Do you think his new parents know what to do for him when he cries?"

"I'm sure they do, honey. Usually all the baby needs is to be fed, burped or a diaper changed. It's pretty easy."

"Do you have a baby? Is that why you know all these things?"

"No. I used to babysit my brother's two boys when they were babies."

Jan sat her in the chair and handed her a handkerchief to blow her nose while she made her bed.

Melinda asked Jan if she was married, and Jan told her she was engaged. Then Melinda looked very thoughtful as she asked, "Have you ever had sex?"

"No, Melinda, I haven't."

"Did any guy ever try to have sex with you?"

"Only once, while at a drive-in movie theater. I was dating one of the star football players, and he became very aggressive. When I said no, he wouldn't stop, so I took my high heeled shoe off and hit him with it, jumped out of the car and started to run home. As luck would have it, a friend of my brother's stopped and gave me a ride home. He wanted to go back and beat up the guy, but I don't think he did. I guess the word got around, and I was never bothered again."

Melinda smiled and said, "Now, you're my hero."

Jan enjoyed postpartum even though she was anxious to move on to more exciting territory. It wasn't long before she was back in labor and delivery. She walked in to an empty nurses station, where the phone was ringing off the hook. She picked up the receiver and said, "Labor and Delivery. This is Miss Winston. May I help you?"

An admitting clerk on the other end said, "I have an orderly bringing a lady up who is in labor. Will you please admit her?"

Jan answered "yes" when the elevator dinged and an orderly came through the double doors. He said, "She tells me she feels like pushing, so I think we'd better get her into bed right away."

Jan ran with him to the nearest room and they helped her into bed as she told Jan, "Honey, this is my sixth baby, and it's moving really fast. I think I may deliver any minute!"

Jan grabbed a "bed delivery pack" just in case, pulling the curtain around so she could check her progress. As the patient spread her legs apart, Jan could see the baby's head crowning. She pushed the emergency call light, opened the delivery pack and the next thing she knew, the patient hollered, "I have to push!"

In a matter of seconds, the baby's head appeared. The patient pushed again and a shoulder appeared, and then the other and out slid the baby. Jan just did what she had previously observed. She cleaned out the baby's mouth as he let out a strong cry, and then she cut the umbilical cord and handed the baby to his mother while she massaged the fundus and waited for the placenta to disengage from the mother's uterus. It took about 10 minutes, and while Jan was waiting, she put the drops in the baby's eyes and took his footprints. Once the placenta was gone, Jan started to clean up the mother.

Just then the curtains parted and there stood Miss Burton and Mrs. Novak. They looked first at Jan, then the baby, then at the mother and back to Jan. They were staring with their mouths wide open. Miss Burton composed herself first and said, "Miss Winston, what have you done?"

Jan laughed out loud. "I've had a baby!"

Mother and nurses laughed with her as Mrs. Novak said, "So you have. Yes you have!"

Jan giggled more and said to the mother, "And I don't even know your name."

Mrs. Novak looked at Jan and said, "You'd better cover your uniform with a smock or you will scare other patients half to death! We'll take over from here."

Jan looked down at her apron and it was covered with blood. She hurried to get a smock.

Two more calls came in with mothers in labor. Jan admitted them, and she was able to assist the doctor with another birth in the delivery room.

* * *

Frank had been transferred to the fifth floor for physical therapy in orthopedics, so Jan went to find him there. She hurried because she was now back to college classes in the afternoon. She found him in hydrotherapy being pampered with a massage. He saw her and said, "Jan, tell them they have to keep this up all afternoon. It's doctor's orders, right?"

Jan laughed and said, "I really think I should be allowed in there because I have been busy delivering babies all morning." She told him about her morning, and everyone laughed.

She left in a hurry so she could change and meet Allen. She got on the elevator with a couple of other people. They stopped at the fourth floor to get out, and Jan pushed the button to go to the lobby. The elevator shimmied a little, went down a few feet and came to a sudden stop. *Oh, no. What's going on here? Why did the lights go out? I can't see a thing.* The elevator jolted and stopped again, causing serious panic to overwhelm her. She screamed, then breathed rapidly, triggering an episode of hyperventilation! *Am I going to die in this thing? Someone please help me! I'm shaking all over, my heart is throbbing. I feel like I'm going to pass out! Okay, this panic is not going to help me. Get a hold of yourself, and stop this right now.* She took a deep breath, willing herself to calm down. *Somewhere on the panel is an emergency button, if only I can remember where it's located. It's so pitch black in here I can't make out anything, let alone the panel.* Jan slowly waved her hands in front of her. Moving her feet a step at a time until she hit a wall. She felt around for the panel and felt nothing. She began to make her way around the walls, feeling for the panel. *Why am I feeling so disorientated? The elevator seems so much bigger. OH! I feel the doors, the panel is to the left. There it is! Now, which button is the emergency one? I'll just start pushing buttons-one, two, three.* The elevator dropped and trembled. *Oh, my God, it's going to fall. I've heard of that happening. I'm going to be killed!* Her panic returned. She reached into her pocket and unpinned her engagement ring, and slipped it on her finger. *There, I'll die with my ring on so Allen will know how much I loved him. Back to the buttons-four, five. Yes, the bell went off! I'll just keep pushing it over and over again-pushing, pushing. They will rescue me soon, I hope. Please, Lord, let them find me before the elevator drops and I die!*

CHAPTER TWENTY SIX
COMPLETE AND TOTAL PANIC!

Allen kept watching the front door of the dorm, sure that Jan would be coming through it any minute. He got out of the car to stretch and waved to a couple of the students as they came out to catch the bus. He hollered at them, "Hey, have you seen Jan?"

One of them answered, "No, but she might have been held up assisting in a delivery of a baby. She'll probably be out soon."

That's right, she's up there with babies being born. She was so cute as she bubbled with excitement over this assignment. She has probably lost track of time, but she's never been late before. Hope she's alright. Allen decided to make good use of his time, so he went to the back of his car. He pulled the little door open that covered the engine, checked the oil, closed the door, and then took his handkerchief out of his pocket to polish some of the chrome. Meanwhile the bus pulled away.

He looked at the sky as an ominous dark cloud drifted over the sun. Allen was overcome with a really bad feeling. His mouth went dry, his stomach felt twisted and his breathing came in short gasps. Jan was in some kind of trouble. He went to the front door of the dorm and knocked. The housemother greeted him. "Hi Allen. What's up?"

"Could you check and see if Jan's in her room. She's never this late, and I'm worried about her."

"Sure, no problem." She turned and went up the stairs.

Coming back down, Allen could see a concerned look on her face. "Not a sign of her and her books are sitting on her desk."

Allen was more concerned than he wanted to reveal. He calmly said, "If she comes back to the dorm, please tell her I'll be right back, okay?"

"I sure will, Allen."

* * *

Jan continued to ring the bell at least two dozen times and more, until her finger felt like it was going to fall off. The elevator suddenly gave a quivering jerk, and Jan screamed! In desperation she held her finger on the bell until she couldn't stand it any longer. Her knees were starting to shake, and she began to tremble all over, so she slid down the wall and sat on the floor. *I'll pound on the doors-bang, bang, bang, I don't have the strength to do it. I feel like I'm going to throw up.*

I'll just make believe Allen is here with me. He would protect me. Maybe if I curl up in a ball and hold my head, I won't die when it hits bottom. Oh, Allen, I wish you were here! He's waiting for me. He'll find me. He'll rescue me. I'm so sleepy! Time dissolved for her. There was no beginning or end. *I can't think. Where's my mind? I need to pound on the door again. I can't move. I'm so hot and sweaty and thirsty. Is someone going to bring me some water? I hear a noise. Oh, it must be Allen. He'll bring me a nice, cold glass of water. I can't keep my eyes open, I'm so sleepy.*

* * *

Allen ran to the hospital, taking the front steps two at a time and ran to the elevators where he pounded on the doors and rang the bells one after the other. He toyed with the idea of running up the stairs to the fifth floor, but he was pretty sure the elevator would be faster. He waited. Finally one opened, people came out, more entered with him. Finally he reached the fifth floor and hurried down the hall to his dad's room.

"Allen, what are. . ."

"Dad, did Jan come to see you before she left the hospital?"

"Yes, Allen, she did. I was in hydro therapy and she was excited about. . ."

"Dad, think, how long ago was that? When did she leave?"

"Oh, son, that was at least an hour ago, probably more. What's happen. . ."

"Dad, I can't explain. I just have to find her!"

Allen ran back to the elevator. Somehow he knew he had to find out why one of the elevators wasn't working. There must be a connection, so he went looking for someone who might know. He stood in front of the working elevators and impatiently waited for one to return to the fifth floor. When it came, he took it to the fourth floor. Stepping out, he looked around and saw nothing. He asked a few nurses who walked by but they didn't know why it wasn't working.

He pushed the button again and waited. Stepping on, he went to the third floor and exited again. There he saw a maintenance man. "Sir, do you know anything about the elevator that's out of operation?"

"No, I just know it's stuck between floors, and they're working on it one floor down."

"Thanks," Allen said as he flew to the stairs and ran down to the second floor. Three men were working feverishly. They were looking up at the bottom of the elevator that was stuck, trying to restart it and bring it down.

Allen walked up, trying to keep his voice calm. "Do you know if anyone is in the elevator you're working on?"

The men looked at him suspiciously. "Why are you asking?"

"My fiancée is missing and she would have been coming down the elevator about an hour and a half ago."

"Well, sir, I have no idea who's in the elevator, but we do know that someone's in it because they rang the emergency bell several times until just recently."

"How soon do you think you can get it open?"

"I wish we knew."

"Is there air circulating inside?"

"No, sir. Not with the power out."

Allen felt a cold sweat develop on his brow as his body moved like a robot ready to disintegrate into a million pieces! He imagined her suffering from an absence of oxygen, struggling to breath, or worse yet, not breathing at all. He felt like a wild man ready to pounce on these useless men making little to no effort. He wanted to tear them apart to get them to take drastic actions to rescue his beloved Janet. He could not lose her now. He looked at their useless efforts; fighting against an overwhelming sense of rage!

"Isn't there a door on the top of the elevator?" He cried.

"Yes, but it's between floors, and we can't get to it."

Suddenly the elevator jerked down and shook like a wet dog.

Allen screamed, "Do something NOW. My fiancée could die in there. Get the door open. Help her, you idiots!" Allen moved toward them like an enraged animal.

CHAPTER TWENTY SEVEN
AT PEACE IN A FIELD OF WILDFLOWERS

Thoughts bounced around Allen's head like a ping pong ball gone wild! He felt terror, frustration and aggravation all jumbled together. He could barely clear his thoughts enough to take a breath. While pacing back and forth like a mad man, a voice broke into his anguished thoughts. It was a female voice. Whirling around, he stood staring at a nurse dressed in white. His mind attempted to focus through his blur of emotions. He glanced down at her name tag, "Mrs. Novak" sounded familiar.

"Hello Allen, I met you in the hall a while back, I'm Mrs. Novak. When I realized it may be Miss Winston in the elevator, I took the liberty of calling the fire department. They should arrive any minute to assist in the rescue."

Allen wanted to cry and hug this nurse all at the same time. "Oh, thank you so much. I'm frantic with worry! She's been in there for about an hour and a half without any circulating air. I'm not sure if anyone can survive that long without air. I'm petrified right now!"

Just then they heard voices, and some firemen stepped out of an elevator, while two stayed on the elevator to go up to the next floor. The fire chief walked over to them. "Do you know who called the fire department?"

Mrs. Novak didn't hesitate to answer, "I did."

"You did the right thing. You said this person has been in there close to two hours?"

Allen answered, "By my calculations, a little over an hour and thirty minutes without air."

The fire chief looked at Allen. "And you are?"

"I'm her fiancé."

"Whose fiancé?"

"The student nurse in that elevator."

"Okay, thank you, sir. He turned his attention to Mrs. Novak. "I just want to find out why we weren't called earlier!"

Mrs. Novak answered. "The maintenance men might be able to answer your question. I just took matters into my own hands."

He turned to one of the maintenance men. "Who is your supervisor and where can I find him?"

One of the men mumbled, "Probably in his office."

"Would you notify your supervisor that I want to talk to him immediately!"

One of them headed for the stairs, while the other stepped back out of the way.

Allen was vaguely aware of a crowd gathering as Mrs. Novak remained at his side. They could hear noises from the shaft, and suddenly the elevator started inching its way down to the second floor. As they watched, he felt severed from reality. He didn't have any desire to be there when they brought her out. He couldn't survive anything drastic happening to her. The thought brought a stabbing pain to his heart. His throat shut off his air, and he wanted to sink to his knees and wail like a wounded animal. His world, his desire for living, would fall into a deep cavern with no way out!

Slowly the elevator was in place, and a couple of firemen were pulling the door apart. As he stared inside, all he could see were the backs of two men in their dark blue uniforms hunched over, doing something with Jan. He could see her white stockings and the hem of her uniform. He thought he could see blood stains on it. Allen wanted to scream, "Is she alright?" He felt his tears without feeling his sobs.

He no longer felt his heart beating, as if he was in a state of suspended animation. Someone came around the corner with a gurney, and one of the firemen reached down to cradle her in his arms.

***

I feel weightless, surrounded by a field of wildflowers. What a delightful perfume they have. I want to run in the wonderful fresh air. I want to breath it in, why is it so hard to breath? My lungs won't let me breath. Allen is kneeling down beside me. I feel his gentle kiss. I'm encompassed by a kaleidoscope of bright colors-blue, green, gold, red. There is an even brighter white light behind them. What are the strange noises around me-banging, buzzing. Stop the noise. Leave me alone! I just want to sleep among the flowers with Allen beside me. Why are people hollering and someone is touching me. They're putting something on my face. Go away, I'll scream. Nothing's coming out. Why can't I fight them off? Why can't I move?

Suddenly she breathed in the fresh air. Her eyes flew open. *The light is so bright, it's hurting my eyes! I'm floating in air, hearing voices. Someone's leaning over me. I can't seem to focus, to see who it is. I see his eyes. It's my Allen, and he's crying! I'll lift my arm and put it around his neck. It won't work. What's happened to me? I'm seeing flashes from cameras, why are they taking my picture? I just want Allen. Where did he go? Why is a doctor examining me? Mrs. Novak has her face close to me. She's talking to me.*

"Jan, it's alright honey, you were stuck in the elevator for a very long time and the doctor wants to see how you're doing. Allen's right here with you. He will hold your hand in just a minute, okay?"

Jan began to remember *pushing buttons, darkness, couldn't breathe.* She felt Allen's hand reach for hers and a sense of calm transferred as if they were aware of each other. As long as he was there she knew everything was alright. The doctor had been checking her reflexes and asking her questions. She tried to think, but everything was lost in a blur of confusion.

The doctor leaned down close to her ear. "It's alright, Janet. I'm going to write some orders and be back to check on you in a minute. Don't fight the oxygen mask. You need to keep it on."

Jan tried to focus on the doctor. Attempting to talk, but the words were held captive somewhere inside her tongue. It was so frightening!

From the moment Allen saw Jan, he knew she must be in pretty bad shape. He wanted to ask why her apron was so bloody, but decided to wait until later. He was overwhelmingly grateful she was alive, but she seemed so out of it. Allen was frightened. He whispered to Mrs. Novak, "Is she going to be alright? She's acting so strange, and it's scaring me!"

"Allen, it's going to take awhile for her to come around. In the meantime, just let her rest. You can use the phone to call her parents or anyone else you think should be notified."

Allen saw an older, very tall, dark-haired nurse standing at the door.

Mrs. Novak spoke up. "Hello, Miss Kingston. Please come in."

Miss K. walked past Allen to Mrs. Novak. "How is she?"

"We think she'll be fine with a little time. She was in the elevator a very long time with the power off."

"Can you stay with her?"

"Of course!"

"Please page me if anything changes." She turned to go. "I'm sorry, I walked right by you young man. Are you a relative of Miss Winston's?"

"Well, yes, sort of. Actually Miss Kingston, I'm her fiancé."

"Oh, I didn't know. When do you intend to get married?"

"As soon as possible after graduation."

"Well, in that case, I wish you well."

Jan appeared to be sleeping, so he dialed her parents, not sure how to approach the subject. He waited, trying to gather his composure in spite of his heart pounding to the beat of a jack hammer. It rang several times, Finally her father answered, "Hello, this is the Winston residence."

Allen tried to calm the tremor in his voice. "Hello, Bill. This is Allen, and I have some news about Jan."

"My goodness, is she alright?"

"She's sleeping right now. She was stuck in the hospital elevator for about an hour and a half with no power or air circulating."

"Oh my goodness! Has she been able to talk to you?"

"No, her head has been in a fog so far, but she's breathing in oxygen with a mask, and they are giving her fluid with an IV."

"Allen, we're coming right down!"

"You may want to wait for a little bit, see how she is when she wakes up."

"No, we need to be there. We'll see you in a few hours or so."

"Okay, see you then."

"Mrs. Novak, I think I'll run upstairs to tell my folks and. . ."

"You won't have to son. We tracked you down."

Allen turned around to see his mom pushing his dad in a wheelchair. "How is she son?"

"We're playing the waiting game at the moment. Mrs. Novak, I'd like you to meet my parents, Carmela and Frank Morris."

"Are you her nurse?" Frank asked.

"You might say so. I'm really one of her instructors just waiting here with Allen to see how things go."

"How bad was she?"

"She hasn't been able to talk much yet, and she's pretty exhausted. We assume it was a major ordeal she went through."

"Thank you, Mrs., what was it? Novak or Nowak?"

"Novak will do just fine."

Allen went back to the phone, calling the nurse's dormitory. The housemother answered. Allen said, "Hi, this is Allen and I thought I'd better bring you up to date on Jan."

"Oh, thank you for calling. I've been worried sick. Where did you find her?"

Allen filled her in on the events and told her he would let her know of future developments. He then left the room in search of more chairs to accommodate everyone. When he returned, Jan was awake.

"Hi, Pumpkin. How's my sweetheart?"

Jan looked at him with a weak smile and touched his hand with hers. Then she reached up and stroked his cheek. Her face contorted into a grimace as she grabbed the mask and pulled it off.

"Jan, honey, you need that on. . ."

Mrs. Novak intervened at Allen's side. "It's okay, let's leave it off for a moment and see if she can talk. Do you hurt anywhere, Jan?"

She stared first at Allen and then at Mrs. Novak and shook her head "no."

"Okay, do you remember what happened in the elevator?"

She shook her head "yes."

"Can you tell us about it?"

Jan stared at Allen for a few moments and then slowly articulated, "You . . . kissed . . . me."

Mrs. Novak asked her, "Did he kiss you in the elevator?"

Allen whispered, "I wasn't in the elevator."

"It's okay, so Allen helped you in the elevator?"

Jan shook her head "yes."

"Okay, that's enough for now. We better keep the mask on for awhile longer."

Janet drifted off to sleep holding Allen's hand.

They quietly talked for awhile, then the doctor came in. "Has she been awake?" he asked, looking at Mrs. Novak. She told him what Jan said, and he looked at Allen. "That's a good sign. Now if you all would step out of the room for a minute, I'd like to do some tests on her. Nurse Novak, please stay."

CHAPTER TWENTY EIGHT
THE KISS IN THE ELEVATOR

The doctor did a full range of neurological tests to which Jan responded well. Before the doctor left, he stopped in the hall and told Allen, "She's making good progress, considering what she went through. I'd say she'll make a full recovery. I'll come by in the morning, and I'd guess by then she'll be able to return to her normal schedule."

Allen walked back into the room. "Mrs. Novak, I'm so grateful you called the fire department when you did." He sat down, putting his head in his hands, and said a quick, silent prayer of gratitude.

His mom hugged him and said, "I'm going to take your dad to his room, and I'll be back later to meet Jan's parents, okay?"

"Of course, Mom, and thank you."

Jan was sound asleep with a tight grasp holding Allen's hand. He wasn't about to leave her room until he knew that she had completely recovered. He looked at her beautiful face and became overwhelmed with the reality of what she meant to him. He thought about the fireman saying the elevator was hanging by a thread. He could not twist his mind around the possibility of losing her permanently. He felt a powerful sense of joy.

Early that evening her parents arrived. After greeting them, he filled them in on all the details as well as the encouraging words of the doctor.

Bill asked, "When you called, did you know the imminent danger she was in?"

"No, I found that out later. It's a miracle that she survived. I credit Mrs. Novak for doing what should have been done much earlier."

Mrs. Novak gently put her hand on Allen's arm. "It just seemed to be the logical action to take."

Bill spoke to Mrs. Novak. "It sounds to me like you were her guardian angel!"

"Thank you, and since you're here to watch over her, this angel is going to fly home to her little angels at home. Nice meeting everyone, and I'll be back first thing in the morning."

Allen looked up, saying, "Thanks, I'll be right here when you return."

Allen visited with Jan's folks, telling them the news of their engagement, when his Mom walked in.. Allen introduced her, "Mom, I'd like you to meet Bill and Muriel Winston. This is my Mom, Carmela Morris."

They all sat down and Muriel and Carmela immediately started talking about the news of the engagement. They discussed having bridal showers in their home towns. As they talked, Jan began to stir, getting more and more restless.

Jan's mom got up from her chair. "Allen, is she alright?"

Jan opened her eyes and looked at Allen. "I need, I have to, please get a nurse."

Jan's mom started to go out just as three student nurses showed up at the door.

Mandy reached her first as Allen said, "She's asking for a nurse."

"That would be all of us. Let me talk to her. Jan, its Mandy, what do you want?"

"I have to pee!"

Cindy turned to Allen and the parents. "Would you step out for a minute?"

As they left, the girls closed the door and helped Jan.

Janet giggled a little about using a bedpan, and when she was finished she grabbed Mandy's hand and said, "Please stay. She looked at Cindy and Kim. Would you all stay?"

They fussed over her, fixing pillows and straightening sheets. Kim took a comb out of her pocket and smoothed her hair. Cindy put some lipstick on her, and then Mandy gave her a drink.

She basked in the attention, and then she said, "Thanks. You are all wonderful."

When Jan's folks walked in, she stared at them. "I didn't know you where here," as she started to cry.

Her dad leaned over her and said, "We came down to play in the elevator with you."

She put an arm around his neck, kissed him on his cheek and murmured, "Okay."

Allen told the girls more about what had happened, and they were astounded at the condition of the elevator and the way she was found. He also mentioned the bloody apron.

Mandy was holding her hand as she quipped, "She must be doing okay because she's cutting off the circulation to my hand!" She stepped over to the bag of Jan's clothes, pulling out the apron. "I'd take a wild guess that she delivered a baby."

"You really think so?" Allen asked.

Mandy held the apron in front of Janet. "Can you tell me how your apron got all bloody?"

Jan stared at the apron for a long time. Then she blurted out, "Oh, I remember! I delivered a baby in bed that couldn't wait for the delivery room."

Everyone laughed at her reaction. Then her parents said they were tired, and would be staying at their cousins. They promised to be back in the morning.

The girls visited for awhile before they went back to the dorm. Jan had gone back to sleep, and Allen stayed in her room.

Jan woke up a couple of hours later and said, "My head hurts. Can you get the nurse?" They brought her a couple of aspirin. When Jan was sound asleep again, Allen went over to a more comfortable chair, laying his head back to sleep.

When Allen woke up in the morning, he went to the restroom to wash his face and hands. When he returned, Jan was sitting up, and he asked, "Do you remember anything?"

Answering with her normal enthusiasm, she said, "Most of it, but it's more like a horrible nightmare than reality. From now on, I'm taking the stairs. Even if it's the Empire State building." Then she looked at him and asked, "How did you know it was me in the elevator?"

"Well, I ran into a phone booth, tore off my shirt, and emerged as Superman! Then I flew down the elevator shaft. Using my x-ray vision, I looked through the steel wall and found you lying on the floor. So I punched a hole in the wall and rescued you."

"Oh, Allen! Now tell me the real story."

"Pumpkin, when the firemen reached you, they said you had passed out."

"But Allen, you were inside the elevator with me."

"No, I was standing outside, but never in there with you."

"I'm not kidding. I was thirsty, and I couldn't breathe. You were beside me and kissed me."

"We didn't know you got in the elevator with her." Jan's mom said as they walked in.

"No, really I wasn't!" Allen said forcefully.

Jan turned in the bed toward her folks. "He was there! I was in this field of wildflowers and Allen, you knelt down beside me and kissed me. I felt you kiss me. I know you were there with me!"

Jan's mom moved over next to Allen. "It's just possible you were part of her miracle survival."

"When you put it that way, maybe I was."

"I know you were!" Jan said in such a way, he had to believe.

The doctor came in to check on her, "I'm going to release you and allow you to go back to the nurses' dorm.

Jan looked at him and said, "Not until you give me something to eat. I'm starved."

Her folks stayed awhile longer, and then left for home. Allen walked her back to the dormitory. He agreed to come back after a shower and some rest to join her for lunch at the cafeteria then drive her to college. As the other students saw them come in for lunch, they jumped up to hug her and tell her how happy they were she was okay. The girls asked them to join their table so they could hear all about her ordeal. Jan and Allen got their food and sat down to tell their stories. Allen had to get a laugh by telling his Superman tale, and the girls were totally entertained.

***

Jan continued to enjoy her "minute of fame." She could hardly believe it when her picture appeared the next day on the front page of the local paper. She looked dead as the firemen lifted her onto the gurney. She realized then what an impact that must have had on Allen to see her like that.

His emotions probably dropped into the depths of the ocean floor. Everybody in the hospital was talking about it. Even in her college classes, they were amazed to see her back on her feet. She kept a copy of the newspaper for posterity-something to show her grand kids.

***

Thursday night, Jan and Allen went to Carol's for dinner. She had fried chicken, mashed potatoes and gravy topped off with corn on the cob. They talked about everything from politics to their engagement. As they walked out the door, Carol said to Jan, "You'll have to answer to me if you don't marry him, my little one!"

"Don't worry, we're already attached at the hip!"

CHAPTER TWENTY NINE
A DIRE PREDICTION

Back in labor and delivery, Jan became quite the expert at delivering babies. Sometimes they would get a mother into the delivery room, and the doctor wouldn't show up in time. So guess who did the delivery? Miss Burton let Jan have the experience each time.

One mother was admitted in labor, carrying twins. She was extremely obese, adding to the size of her already huge belly. Dr. Christensen came in to examine her, saying, "Looks like you're coming along very well. I'll have the nurse bring in the paper for you to sign to do the Cesarean Section."

The mother answered, "I've decided I don't want you to do that. Surgery is against our religion and I will have them by natural childbirth."

Jan could tell the doctor was struggling with this as he calmly answered, "Mrs. Nielsen, I explained why you would need the Cesarean in my office, and you agreed. What has changed your mind?"

"I talked it over with my husband and some people in my church, and they advised me not to allow it."

The father, who was sitting in a chair across the room, spoke up, "Did you hear my wife, we don't believe in surgery, she has made up her mind and you will deliver these babies like any other delivery."

"Sir, that would be fine if your wife were a normal weight and this were a single birth. I will not be held responsible for allowing a natural delivery because most likely one or more of them will not survive due your wife's extreme obesity."

"We have made our decision. My wife will not have surgery."

Jan had assisted Dr. Christensen many times, and he was a great doctor-always calm, encouraging his mothers, with a good sense of humor. Anger was so unlike him. He turned toward the father, and in a stern voice said, "Sir, I need to talk to you in private. Follow me to the conference room."

In the meantime, the mother's contractions were increasing, while the nurses thought they might have to deliver the twins in bed.

They could hear shouted words emanating through the hall from the conference room, and suddenly Dr. Christensen flew out the door. He tore by the nurses' station and entered the mother's room. He talked to her in the tone of an angry father to his rebellious teenager. "You need to listen to me and hear me out before you say a word. You are extremely overweight. If you insist upon delivering these babies by natural childbirth, you are most likely going to cause their death and could very well cause your own as well When we talked about this in my office, you agreed to surgery. I don't know what or who has changed your mind, but ultimately the decision is yours. Give me permission to do the cesarean, and we will prep you immediately."

"No, I already told you, it's against my religion!"

The doctor slapped the bedside stand with his hand. "So you want to kill your babies and very

possibly yourself as well?"

The mother sobbed, "My husband said, God will help us survive. I will not be cut open with your knife!"

He stomped out of the room, going down to the nurses' station grabbing the phone as he dialed a number. "Yes, is the chief in? Okay, will you page him STAT to labor and delivery?" He then called the hospital attorney. "Hello, Ned. This is Samuel, and I need a favor STAT. I need a form stating in your legal language that the parents of unborn twins will not hold the doctors or the hospital responsible for their personal decision to have natural childbirth against my advice. I need it signed before delivery, like in the next 15 minutes. Can you do that for me? Thanks, Ned. I owe you one."

Dr. Hancock, Chief of Obstetrics, walked in. "What's up Sam?"

"Let's go into the conference room." As they walked off together, Dr. Christensen said to Miss Burton, "I pray that we can all survive what we are about to witness in the next hour or so."

The nurses looked at each other as Miss Burton turned to Jan calmly. "Miss Winston, would you go and check the mother's progress and report back to me?"

When Jan opened the door, a man in a tailored suit was at the patient's bedside explaining a document to the couple. He then asked them to sign. *Obviously he's the lawyer. He wasted no time getting here.* The mother shakily took the pen while moaning in pain and signed. Her husband stepped up quickly and did the same.

Jan asked the father to leave, and after examining the mother, she went back to report, "She's nine centimeters dilated and 100% effaced. It shouldn't be much longer."

"Okay, let's get her to the delivery room."

Jan went back, and the doctors walked in behind her. At that moment, the patient loudly moaned in severe pain. Dr. Hancock stepped up without introducing himself and examined her. He then said to her, "I am Dr. Hancock, the chief of obstetrics, and I completely agree with Dr. Christensen. I see no possible way that you can deliver these twins alive through a normal delivery. There is nothing normal about this, and you are definitely risking the lives of your babies, as well as your own. Won't you please reconsider, and we will swiftly take you to surgery before it is too late?"

She let out a lengthy scream and hollered, "NO!"

Jan and Miss Burton took her down and prepared her for delivery. Jan thought *Please let the doctors be wrong this time. Please let the mother and babies survive.* The mother was so overweight that she could barely lift her tremendous bulk onto the delivery table. Each side of her buttocks and back draped over the table. Her enormous arms hung over with no room left to rest them beside her. Her breathing came in short gasps. The doctors could not offer an epidural due to her obesity, they proceeded with coaching her in delivery. She was pushing until she was blue in the face and the baby's head would not crown. Jan thought, *Oh no, the doctor's predicted a problem giving birth naturally, and it appears they may have been right.* They went ahead and did an episiotomy on each side of the birth canal without asking permission, knowing she would refuse. Jan was waiting for a baby's head to appear, but it just didn't happen.

Suddenly, one of the docs went up to her abdomen and pushed with all of his weight at the same time that she pushed, and the other doctor reached up into the birth canal with an instrument trying to pull a baby out. They continued this for each contraction. After several minutes a head started to crown! Jan was so excited to finally see it. Slowly the baby inched its way out. Its head was elongated and as it appeared Jan noticed that its skin looked like crinkled wax paper. She instinctively knew it must be dead. The doctor handed her the baby, saying, "He's been dead for awhile; this is pathetic!" Jan walked over to the bassinet and carefully placed the baby in it.

The mother had very little strength left to do anything. Jan noticed that her skin tone was turning a chalky color. She went around to the mother's side, put her stethoscope up to her ears and pumped up the extra large blood pressure cuff that was already on her arm. Jan struggled to hear and immediately turned to the doctors and said, "It's 42 over 0, barely audible!"

Dr. Christensen took in a deep breath and said, "Oh, my God. We're going to lose her too!"

They shouted at her to take a breath. Dr. Hancock hit her chest, but she was no longer responding.

Meanwhile the doctors worked to pull the other baby out, hoping that they could at least save one of the twins. They worked and worked. Finally the baby's head emerged, and it was very obvious that Doctor Christensen's devastating prediction had come true. We had lost all three! Jan took the twin and placed him next to his brother. She wanted to drop to her knees and weep, but she held her emotions in check and began the cleanup.

Both doctors complimented the nurses and thanked them for all of their help. Doctor Hancock stood shaking his head while Doctor Christensen took his smock off, slamming it to the floor, his voice quivering with grief. "Damn it, why wouldn't they listen? And what do you want to bet when I tell her husband, he will blame me or his wife?"

The doctors left together, and as they went out the door, Miss Burton said, "We'd better clean them up right away in case the father comes in for a viewing."

Jan had already started with the babies, cleaning their little bodies and placing them on a clean sheet. She took a clean blue receiving blanket out and covered them up to their faces, noticing how peaceful they looked.

There was no way that the nurses could move the mother, but they cleaned all around her, took her legs out of the stirrups, bringing the table up and laying her flat. She was clean, and Jan put a new white sheet over her body.

They were ready to take the refuse out when Doctor Christensen walked in with the father and the hospital chaplain. Jan slid the garbage over in the corner and stood quietly in front of it. The father went over to the twins first and broke down sobbing. He turned on his heel and went to stand beside his wife's body. He said, "Why didn't you have enough faith that He would protect you?"

That was the final word to explode the steam from his pressure cooker. Dr. Christensen turned a bright shade of red and retorted in anger, "These deaths have nothing to do with your wife's faith, but it was your distorted beliefs that created this catastrophe! I am seriously considering bringing charges against you for murder in the first degree! Now go to the nurses' station and make arrangements for the bodies then leave our hospital immediately!"

The Chaplain ushered the father out the door, Jan heard Chaplain Russell say, "The Lord uses educated people with the knowledge to advise us in complicated situations such as this. He works through them to bring about His good works, your wife is not responsible!"

As the door shut, the nurses clapped for Dr. Christensen.

* * *

Miss Burton called for four strong orderlies to move the heavy body to the morgue while Jan carried the babies down herself before getting ready for class.

When she went to lunch, she broke down and cried as she told the other nursing students the events of her morning. This was their day to attend nursing classes in their own classroom. Miss Kingston asked her to repeat what happened. It brought up many questions regarding religious and cultural practices within the hospital.

It brought laughter when Mandy asked about the foreign family who brought in a dead chicken dripping blood, and wanted to hang it over the bed of their mother. While some customs were to be honored, something like that could not be allowed because of possible disease.

The tragedy of the morning ended with some very stimulating learning.

Jan was so glad this occurred on a day when she didn't see Allen. She would not want to share her emotional state with him. It was something that would not be shared with anyone except her colleagues.

The memories of that tragic day slowly faded as Jan shared the joy of bringing new life into the world on a daily basis. She observed there were all kinds of mothers in labor. Many endured their pain in steadfast stoic silence. Some cussed at their husbands, and a few screamed from the beginning to the end, sharing with everyone within earshot. But every mother melted with pure delight as she cuddled her newborn infant. Jan became determined, when it was her turn to experience childbirth, she would join the ranks of those who endured quietly. She realized she had no idea what labor was really like. For her remaining time in labor and delivery, she would walk out those double doors gliding on cloud nine.

CHAPTER THIRTY

TO THE RESCUE

Jan's next rotation was the pediatric ward, which brought back many memories of the children's home. She saw the familiar cribs, feeling as if she had come home. As Jan walked by the rooms, she heard a child's voice hollering out, "I gotta piss!" She saw the child jumping up and down in his crib, while holding on to his dinker with all his might.

At that same moment, she saw Miss Page enter the room with a urinal. She waited until the child was finished and Miss Page was able to greet her. "Well, hello, Miss Winston."

Jan was enthusiastic about being with Miss Page. "This is great to work with you again," said Jan. "it's been almost two years since you were my instructor back in surgery."

"Likewise, Miss Winston."

They walked around in different areas, then stopped for a minute in the middle of the hall while Miss Page explained something to Jan. There was a little boy coming down the corridor who Jan could have sworn had facial hair and a mustache. He came closer, Miss Page said to him in a stern voice, "You behave yourself, Edward!"

Jan thought to herself That's not very nice. He isn't doing anything wrong! He watched Miss Page as he stayed close to the wall, going around them. Suddenly Jan felt her skirt go up from behind, and a hand touched her bottom. She let out a yelp as she jumped sideways, just in time to see Miss Page grab Edward's hand and march him down the hall.

As her instructor came back, she said, "Come into the chart room. I need to explain his behavior." Once they were inside, she reached for Edward's chart and they sat down together. "He suffers from 'Precocious Puberty' which is a disease that brings on early puberty; in Edward's case, at age seven. Do you remember studying this in your pediatric class?"

"Yes, I do, but I didn't think I would see it my first day on pediatrics. If I remember correctly there can be different causes-tumors, glandular and a few other rare diseases.""Correct. He's been hospitalized to run several tests and observe his behavior.

The symptoms of this disease in boys are facial, under arm and pubic hair plus enlargement of the penis and increased masculinity. Edward doesn't know how to react to his hormones. He's a little boy in a man's body. He has quite literally driven the nurses crazy."

Jan observed, "This should be one circumstance where we can be allowed to wear pants."

"Yes, if only they made uniforms with pants and a top."

"Miss Page, maybe we should make some, starting a new trend in uniforms. I can see the headlines, 'Nurses Rebel and Refuse to Wear Dress Uniforms.' Oh, wouldn't you just love it?"

"Dream on, Miss Winston. Dream on. It'll probably never happen."

"So how do we handle this little man monster?"

"We obviously can't let him run wild, so we do use discipline as you just observed. It is very difficult because he's really sneaky sometimes, as he was with you. The poor kid is suffering and doesn't understand why."

"Can't they give him something to curb his libido?"

"When they finish the battery of tests, coming up with the definitive cause, they will start treating it. In the meantime, use discipline."

"Well, I know I'll be watching him like a hawk from now on."

They went over to the contagious disease section and Miss Page gave her a review of the proper procedure; gowns, mask, gloves. "Miss Winston, at the present time we have a couple of cases of meningitis, one staphylococcal pneumonia and one aspiration pneumonia. I would like you to study the charts of these children and the techniques of their care."

"Of course, Miss Page." Jan said.

"Tomorrow and the rest of the week they will be your assignment. Do you feel comfortable using isolation technique?" Miss Page asked.

"It doesn't bother me at all, I've used this technique in other areas of the hospital. The only thing that's different is the age of the patients." Jan answered.

"These children range in age from six months to five years old, and I'm confident you'll do fine Miss Winston."

* * *

Jan missed seeing her future father-in-law after classes. She had been able to develop a remarkable relationship with him, and she now understood why Allen was such a wonderful man. She was so relieved he was no longer snorkeling in the bottom of a whiskey bottle. Jan had been touched with his emotional farewell when he was released to go home on Sunday. "Nurse Jan, I'm going to miss your daily visits. I couldn't love you more if you were my own daughter. He had turned to Allen and admonished, take good care of her and don't ever let her get on the elevator again!"

Between their studies and Allen's work at the station, they only saw each other for a quick meal and a ride to school during the week. Saturday evening came around and they had planned a date. Allen was picking her up in a few minutes to take her to a local concert.

"I don't think I've ever told you how my Dad used to take Mom and I to concerts while I was a teenager." Jan said as they rode in the car.

"So does that mean you enjoy concerts?"

"Yes, I usually do, unless it's a screechy soprano."

"Well, my dear, you're in for a treat, tonight's a band concert."

"Oh, I'll love that." Jan said as they walked into the auditorium.

They sat holding hands, as the music started. About half way through the performance, a man about three rows behind started making rude remarks. His speech was slurred, and even from the distance they could smell alcohol. After a few really demeaning remarks about women, Allen turned in his seat and said, "Would you mind keeping your words to yourself, sir."

"Hey, you up front, if you don't like what I'm saying, come back here, and I'll give you a little drink to calm your nerves."

Allen ignored him and tried to listen to the music again. Jan just sat looking straight ahead, hoping the guy would pass out.

Suddenly from the back the man hollered, "Hey, you, young punk, I was talking to you! Don't you have any manners, or does that sweet little harlot next to you have you all hot and bothered?"

Jan had never seen Allen so mad. She thought he was going to burst when he reared up from his seat, went up the aisle, reached in where the guy was sitting, and pulled him up by his coat. The audience gave some cheers as Allen held him suspended like a rag doll with his feet dangling in air. Jan noticed a couple of other strong men stand up to follow Allen and offer support.

She then heard some angry words from Allen and a door slamming. The three men then came quietly back down the aisle. The audience clapped for them as they returned to their seats. Putting his arm around Jan, he said, "Nobody talks to my special lady that way and gets away with it!"

Jan felt like she was Cinderella rescued by her Prince Charming!

* * *

Jan soon learned that little children on the pediatric floor would always respond to love when crying in pain or frightened. All she had to do was wrap them in her arms and sit quietly with them. She also found them very eager to learn and cooperate if she explained exactly what she was going to do to them. She recognized that if she gave them a choice of being very still on their own or having someone hold them still for an injection or a procedure, they would usually choose to do it themselves. They had remarkable control when given an option. Children were also resilient and bounced back from a painful procedure very quickly.

It continued to bother Jan when parents were told to leave the room when anything was done for their child. She made a commitment to herself that she would implement change, once she graduated and had passed state boards.

* * *

When the students went to their nursing classes at the hospital, Miss Kingston made an exciting announcement.

"The senior class is invited to the annual Christmas hospital staff party. It is on Saturday, December 19, in a little over a month. You may bring one guest, and it's dress-up. It will include dinner and a dance at a large hall downtown." Miss Kingston smiled. "This is their subtle way of recruiting future employees! Any questions? If not, we'll proceed with class."

Jan's mind wandered. What a nice change this will be from our usual dates. I love to dance. I have no clue if Allen likes to dance or if he even knows how. We've never talked about dancing. The subject hasn't surfaced before, but now I can hardly wait to find out. She suddenly heard her name called and realized she had no idea what was being discussed.

She heard Miss Kingston clear her throat and say, "Miss Winston, where has your mind wandered?"

Jan's face flushed as she admitted, "I was already dancing at the party with Allen."

The class roared as Miss Kingston smiled and said, "Well, it's time to excuse yourself from the dance and make your way back to the classroom."

Jan adjusted and said, "I'm sorry Miss Kingston."

Later that afternoon, she tried calling Allen at his room, and then at the gas station. His boss answered, "He's not here right now, he called to say he would be a little late. Something had come up with his Aunt."

Jan immediately called Aunt Barbara and Allen answered. Jan said, "Is Aunt Barbara okay?

"Well, hi, Pumpkin, you tracked me down didn't you? Aunt Barbara's okay. I stopped at my room to change and get rid of my books when she called and said that she had fallen and thought her wrist was broken. I came right over and took her to emergency.

I knew you were in class and I wouldn't be able to call you. She has a small crack in her wrist bone, and he applied a light cast. I just brought her home. What's going on?"

"You're probably in a hurry to get to work, aren't you?"

"I'm never in a hurry when you're on the phone. What's up?"

Jan told him about the party and then asked him if he liked to dance.

"Honey, I struggle to dance. How about you?"

"Oh, sweetheart, I love to dance, and I don't know why we've never talked about it before."

"Well, you're in for a treat, my little chickadee. You can teach me a few steps."

"I can hardly wait. And does that mean we can dance at our wedding?"

"If you don't mind my stepping on your feet."

"Not at all. I step on them too."

"Honey, I hate to end this call, but I really need to get to work, okay?"

"Sure, see you tomorrow."

Jan got off the phone, twirling around as she loudly announced, "I will dance at my wedding."

She paused, "I think."

CHAPTER THIRTY ONE
HER TEMPER FLARES

One morning Jan was assigned a baby born with a severe cleft palate and lip. At first Jan found it difficult to look at him. She held the baby in her arms and as he slept she took the opportunity to study the disfigurement. The middle of the child's top lip was missing, and there was a gaping hole where the roof of his mouth should have been that exposed the inside of his nose. From reading his history, the parents, after seeing their baby, left the hospital and wanted nothing to do with him. The baby awoke, looked at Jan with his big round dark brown eyes, and she cuddled him now that she had moved past his looks. She knew they were doing some experimental surgeries on these children, but it would have to wait until he was older. The most difficult part was trying to feed him. Some babies were able to adapt to a bottle but many required a feeding tube. Miss Page said he would most likely be placed in the Watkins Children's Home.

A few children in this ward had suffered traumatic brain injuries. Most often these injuries were sustained in automobile accidents. As Jan studied the charts and gave different levels of care to each, she was disturbed by the amount of debilitation that occurred from these injuries. These children had severe functional issues. The ages ranged from a few months to ten years old. Most were scheduled for a series of surgeries followed by physical therapy. Jan felt emotionally drained working with these children. The ones in a coma or a semi-comatose state emanated an aura of peace as Jan washed, fed and exercised their frail muscles.

An 18-month-old child had a severe head injury. She was in a depressed level of consciousness with pupil abnormalities, a slow pulse and an elevated blood pressure. While Jan changed her diapers, a couple of doctors walked to her crib.

"I feel she displays classic signs of physical abuse." Doctor Sandretto said.

"You don't think the brain damage is the result of falling from her crib?" Dr. Newberry asked

"No, the bruising to her brain indicates a more severe blow than would occur from a fall and when I talked to the nanny she claims she found the baby un-responsive first thing in the morning after leaving the child in her mother's care for the night."

"So the baby isn't normally in the care of her parents at night?"

"No, and it's just the mother. The nanny told me the mother never cares for her own baby. She was hired to be the sole caregiver."

Dr, Newberry gave the child a thorough exam while Jan assisted him. "Thank you, Miss Winston." he said as he turned toward Dr. Sandretto. "I agree with you Bob, was it your intention to go ahead and call the authorities?"

"Yes, that's why I needed a second opinion."

"I'll back you up Frank."

Jan was horrified by the thought that any parent would physically abuse a beautiful child they'd brought into the world. It was beyond her comprehension, and she found it impossible to imagine. She knew this child had suffered irrevocable pain and damage to her tiny brain, and she just wanted to hold her and love her pain away.

Soon after the doctors left, a woman who looked to be in her 30's approached. She stoically looked down at the child, without any sign of emotion, then turned toward Jan and curtly asked, "What's wrong with her? Why isn't she responding?"

Jan cautiously said, "I'm sorry. I'm not allowed to give out any information about the patients. May I ask if you are a relative or a friend?"

The women snapped, "Yes, I'm her mother, and I need to know what's going on. When my nanny brought her in, she didn't mention she was this bad."

"I understand. Why don't you come with me to the nurses' station and we'll find a doctor to answer your questions."

"I don't want to talk to a doctor; I'm in a hurry to get to work. I'm on my way to court, and I can't be late!"

Jan observed her tailored navy blue suit and high heels. "May I ask why you're going to court?"

The women looked at Jan like she was a total ignoramus. She turned on her heel to leave saying, "I'm a lawyer, and I have a client waiting for me."

As she started for the door, the two doctors were coming back to the room. Jan frantically said, "Doctors, you need to talk to this child's mother." as she made a gesture towards the suspected abused baby.

They acted quickly, positioning themselves in the door while Dr. Sandretto authoritatively said, "Madam, you need to accompany us to the consultation room."

The mother stood her ground with a rebellious voice answering, "I have nothing to say to you, and I must leave immediately to go to court. I'm already late!"

"You're not leaving here until we discuss your child's condition."

She responded with an irritated voice, "If you want answers, I'll bring my nanny in to talk to you. She's responsible for the exclusive care of that child."

The doctors weren't giving up easily as they stood their ground. They persuaded her to come with them for just a few moments. Jan wanted so badly to be able to accompany them. Miss Page came in, and Jan discussed the situation with her.

"Miss Winston, this kind of thing happens more frequently than you want to know. However, it's possible that the mother had nothing to do with it. I'll look into it and see what the outcome is."

Jan later learned that the mother generally worked up to twelve hours a day as a practicing attorney and only saw her child at night when she was sleeping. She had divorced her husband for getting her pregnant and hired a full-time nanny. The nanny was called away on an emergency, and the baby was cranky and disobedient, keeping her mother awake when she had an important case in the morning. The Nanny was willing to testify that the child was non-responsive in the morning when she returned and found her in her crib. The theory was that the mother lost control and somehow incurred a blow to the baby's head which caused a "contrecoup" injury to the brain. (blow to the head severe enough to cause the brain to slam into the other side of the skull, causing an injury on the opposite side.) She was arrested and brought up on child abuse charges. The mother fought it in court, stating that she found the child on the floor in the morning and placed her back in her crib. She theorized the baby climbed over the railing of the crib and fell to the floor. She sent her nanny to emergency with the child. The nanny claimed she hadn't seen the mother that particular morning. Jan found it hard to believe that the mother actually won her case.

Jan also worked with children that had been accidentally poisoned, usually from common household cleaners. This was difficult for Jan as well. Most poisoning could have easily been prevented had the parents been more cautious. Leaving open containers within a child's reach was uncalled for, and yet it was a common occurrence. One-two-year old Jan cared for had swallowed bleach that burned her tongue and throat and ulcerated her esophagus so badly that they had inserted a tube through her abdomen into her stomach to feed her, most likely for the rest of her life.

Jan also worked directly with Miss Page in the pediatric burn unit so she could learn the procedures if she was assigned there as an RN. These children were the most valiant she'd ever cared for. She had a consuming desire to return as a nurse to work with them. She made a note to add that as one of her to-dos should she be able to work at the Watkins Medical Center in the future.

* * *

Allen picked up Jan, as was their regular routine, for lunch and college classes. They laughed and talked over lunch in their favorite ice cream shop when Jan reminded Allen about the hospital dinner and dance coming up on Saturday evening.

Allen looked at Jan with a shocked expression and said, "I thought it was a week from Saturday, and I made plans for us to drive Aunt Barbara up to the folks for an overnight visit. She's so excited about it; I really don't want to break her heart."

Jan's chin fell as she sat there completely speechless.

Allen flippantly said, "It's okay, Pumpkin. There will be other parties to go to. Don't worry about it."

Jan suddenly found her voice and her temper flared as she caustically remarked, "I bought a new dress for this, and I have looked forward to dancing with you for the last month. How could you?"

Allen began to laugh so hard, he could hardly catch his breath as he fanned himself with his napkin. "Whoa, did you really think I would forget an opportunity to hold you in my arms all evening? At least now I know what triggers your temper. I won't be doing that again!"

"Allen, you mean you weren't serious? Now I'm really mad!"

He reached over the table, taking her hands in his and said seriously, "I really thought you would know I was kidding."

Jan could hardly stay mad at him for very long and said weakly, "Allen, I guess I should have known you were kidding, but don't you dare do that to me ever again!"

Allen looked at her with his winning smile and said, "Now, I'd better find a pay phone and tell Aunt Barb the trip is off."

"Allen, that's enough!"

They held hands laughing as they went out the door.

CHAPTER THIRTY TWO
TEACH ME TO DANCE

It was Saturday, Jan's last day in pediatrics. The supervisor asked her to work in the respiratory ward. Of all days for her hair to be exposed to the steam inside the croup tents. It always made her hair look like she'd been playing in the bottom of a fish tank. Children with croup were usually very sick with a characteristic respiration that made a strident, harsh, raspy noise with each breath. The cough sounded like a motorcycle revving its engine with a wasp nest stuck in the tailpipe. She tried to disturb them as little as possible with minimum mouth and body care; any effort on their part to move would bring on their cough.

As she entered the ward, she took off her cap and dressed in the isolation bonnet, gown, mask and gloves. She carefully monitored their IV fluids, checked their temps and gave their medications. This was an acute viral inflammation of the upper and lower respiratory tract. She did not want to spread this virus around. Jan was busy working with a two-year-old victim, when she heard a gurgling sound from across the room. One of the little patients had mucus in his throat, strangling him. She grabbed the suction machine at the same time she pushed the emergency button. She was suctioning when a doctor rushed in. He took over while a nurse said, "It's difficult to save these children when they fill up with so much mucous."

The doctor worked and worked on the three-year-old child to no avail. It was almost more than Jan could bare to see a child die. The doctor finally called the time of his death and said he would notify his parents. Jan knew she would have to do postmortem care on this precious child, and it broke her heart. Death was an integral part of nursing, but she wondered if she would ever get used to it with children.

When it was time to leave, Jan walked down the stairs and forced herself to file her emotions in her back pocket so they would not discolor an evening she envisioned would be filled with the joy of being with Allen and so many of her friends. Since becoming a nurse Jan had become accustomed to doing this. Sharing the downside of the medical profession with anyone not a part of it could easily ruin the mood.

* * *

Mandy was just coming out of the elevator when Jan opened the door of the stairwell. They grabbed each others' hands and as soon as they reached the outdoors, they started running toward the dorm. "Mandy, aren't you glad I talked you into coming to the dance tonight?"

"Honestly, shopping with you and buying new dresses was a lot more fun than sitting and watching everyone dance. In spite of that, I'll be ready in a second, with plenty of time to do your hair and nails."

They went to their separate rooms, took showers and met in Jan's room.

As Mandy started working on her hair, Jan asked, "Mandy, have you ever been on a date?"

"Oh, heavens, no. I was only asked once, and he was the class nerd-short, pimply and fat. He wanted to take me to the prom. I'm not crazy enough about the opposite sex to endure that kind of agony. Besides men always end up being mean to women."

"Oh, my goodness, Mandy, do you think Allen will be mean to me?"

"Oh, no, Jan. Allen's different! He's the most wonderful man I've ever met."

"What about my dad? You've visited with him when they've been here."

"That's true. But what was he like with you and your mom behind closed doors?"

"Oh Mandy, he was a wonderful father to me and a loving husband to my mom."

Mandy got very quiet as she busied herself setting Jan's hair. Jan looked at her in the mirror and was quite sure she was very close to tears.

"Mandy, what is it? You know you can talk to me about anything, and I can tell something is really bothering you."

"Oh Jan, you don't have any idea what it's like to live with a man that's cruel and vicious. My mother, my brother and I have lived in terror all our lives. My mother told me that going to nursing school was my escape and to never ever come back!"

"Oh, honey, what did he do to you?"

In a trembling voice Mandy answered, "It's terribly hard to talk about. In fact, I've never told anyone, and I'm not sure I can."

"It's okay, Mandy, you don't have to tell me if you don't want to."

Mandy was quiet as she finished Jan's hair, pondering whether to speak or not. As she put in the last pin curl, she stood looking at Jan for a very long time before she moved over to sit on the bed. Jan turned her chair around and sat quietly with her hands folded in her lap.

Mandy cleared her throat then looked down at the floor and barely whispered, "He raped me from the time I turned fourteen until I left home."

Jan couldn't speak. She knew this kind of thing happened, but in her wildest imagination she never thought that her dear sweet Mandy would have been a victim. She finally found her voice. "You mean your father did that?"

Mandy shook her head "yes."

"Oh, Mandy, that's terrible. Did you tell your mom or somebody?"

"Jan, my father was an alcoholic. When he drank he was extremely mean. I tried to tell my mother on several occasions, but she always changed the subject. She knew what was going on. I know she did, but she preferred to ignore it. When my brother figured it out, he accosted my dad and screamed at him to stop or he would call the police. My dad beat him really bad and told him he would kill me and our mother if he ever told anyone. My brother left home in the middle of the night the day he turned eighteen, and I'm the only one who knows where he is."

"Mandy, help me to understand. Why does your mother continue to stay with him and why would she allow him to do this to her daughter?"

"I've asked myself those questions many times. I could never understand why she wouldn't help me when I had no one else to turn to. I reflected on all this after starting psychology class. I think I may have figured out some things, but I'm still not sure I really understand."

Jan looked at her with such loving compassion as she said, "Please tell me about it."

"My mother never went to high school. She was forced to get a job as a waitress when she was fourteen to help her family financially. That was how she met my dad. He was nine years older than her and already had a steady job in a large gold mine just outside of town. He was big, strong and really good-looking. She was from a very poor family. He offered her a nice home and a regular income. They got married when she turned 16. I came along four years later when my brother was two. My dad would never let my mom work. He was extremely overbearing and controlling. I think she became very frightened and dependent on him to the point that leaving was not an option. That's why she closed her eyes to the beatings and sexual abuse of herself and her children. She tried to pretend it never happened."

"Mandy, do you ever intend to go back?"

"Absolutely not! I don't really care if I ever see my parents again, but I do want to see my brother."

"Where is he now?'

"Actually, he went to Alaska and works on a fishing boat. I really miss him. We do stay in touch with letters once in a while. I just hope that I can save my money when I start working and go there for a visit."

"Oh, look at the time. Do you want me to do my own makeup?"

"No my dear, you're not going to deprive me of doing something I enjoy! Besides, I don't have much to do to get ready, so let's get busy."

"Mandy, would you like to hitch a ride in Allen's car tonight?"

"Jan, don't you remember the last time I tried to squeeze into his back seat? What a hoot! Besides, I have a ride with a couple of the girls that don't have guests either."

"Okay, that's fine."

***

Jan wiggled into her new, bright red dress and twirled around in front of the mirror. She noticed how the skirt flared out in a circle perfect for dancing-that is, if she could teach Allen how to twirl. She took one last look in the mirror as she grabbed her coat, purse and gloves.

Allen picked her up a little early so they would have plenty of time to talk on their way. They'd been very busy lately making tentative plans for their wedding. Their mothers had already scheduled bridal showers a month apart in April and May. They had picked out a local church with a large reception hall and Allen was going to talk to the preacher next month. It was hard juggling studies and wedding plans at the same time.

They arrived at the party fifteen minutes early and were greeted by the hospital administrator and director of nurses. The band was just starting to set up and the hospital dietary staff was busy decorating the buffet table.

They walked over to a table close to the band and since they were first to arrive, they sat down to talk. Once again, their focus was the wedding. Allen stopped for just a minute and took her hand, saying, "We haven't talked about our honeymoon. Do you have any suggestions?"

The word "honeymoon" brought Jan to the reality that they would no longer be celibate and intimacy would be a large part of their newly married life. She knew she was blushing as she answered, "My only request is to stay away from big cities and enjoy the outdoors. Besides, we can't afford a whole lot until we both start working, right?"

"We seem to be thinking along the same lines, and my folks suggested that we use their cabin isolated high in the mountains. Before you say yes, I have to tell you that it's very primitive. There's no indoor plumbing, there's an outhouse, a pump out front for well water and a very large wash basin big enough for one person to bath in. Oh, and I almost forgot, there's a river we can swim in."

"That sounds wonderful. Can we hike and explore? Will we cook over a campfire? And can we have hot chocolate and marshmallows every night?'"

"We can do all of the above, plus there's an antique wood stove to cook on or heat the cabin. It's really fun, if you like that kind of thing."

"Allen, that sounds like paradise! Will we drive there after the reception?"

"Only if you want to spend most of our wedding night on the road."

"Oh my goodness, how long does it take to get there?"

"About four or five hours. In my little car, probably six."

"Guess we stay in a hotel our first night?"

"Seems that way, and I'll make all the arrangements."

Right about then, the girls arrived, crashing their table, and it looked like the dinner was about to be served. It promised to be a fun night.

※ ※ ※

After a couple of ho-hum talks from the hospital dignitaries giving them time to let their food settle, the band members took their places and started the music. Allen asked Jan if she wanted to dance, and she eagerly stood up. He took her hand and they had barely taken a dance position when he said, "Would you like to show me a few steps? I'm eager to learn."

"Well, of course, my kind sir. Let's start with the basic foxtrot."

She demonstrated and he followed, stumbling a bit. She showed him how to go forward and backward and to each side. Then she asked him if he would like to learn how to twirl her. He was enthusiastic as he said, "Sure."

Once she finished, he asked, "Shall we try it on the dance floor?" Just then the music stopped. They were ready to sit down, and the band started playing another foxtrot. As they approached the dance floor, he asked her, "Are you sure I'm ready for this?"

"Of course, and it's okay if you stumble a bit. I'll catch you."

He took her into his arms, and with a mastery that rocked her off her feet, he danced her around the floor, giving her excellent prompts with his hand on her back, twirling her several times, bringing her to a dipping motion at the end of the song! As he brought her back up, he kissed her quickly and said, "You didn't step on my feet even once."

She looked at him with her eyes bigger than a couple of flying saucers. She shook her head and blurted out, "You can dance!"

Laughing, he said, "Well of course, you're an excellent teacher!"

"Allen, you put me through that whole charade, and you knew how to dance the whole time?"

"Yes, my darling' and wasn't it fun?"

"You've been planning this ever since I told you about the party, haven't you?"

"Planning what?"

"To lie to me and be deceitful and . . ."

"I love it when you're angry."

"Well I don't think it's funny and . . ."

Allen put his arm around her, leading her to the dance floor as the music started, and this time it was a waltz. She looked at him expectantly, and he said, "Don't you want to teach me some of the basics?"

"You're on your own, buster!"

"Okay." He pulled her to him and began waltzing like it was as easy as one, two, three.

When it came to the jitterbug, they had a ball showing off for everyone. They were flabbergasted when people formed a circle around the dance floor just to watch. Jan had never danced with anyone who knew how to dance as well as he did, and it was the most magical event since the first time she laid eyes on him. After several dances, they took a break to drink some punch and sit down with the girls. The nurses couldn't believe they knew how to dance so well. One of the girls blurted out, "You've practiced a lot for this dance, haven't you?"

Allen answered, "No, this was the first time we've ever danced together."

Cindy looked at both of them with a jaundiced eye. "I really find that very hard to believe."

"That's the absolute truth. Didn't you notice that Allen faked me into giving him some lessons?"

"Did you really think he couldn't dance?"

"Oh yeah. He pulled a good one on me, but just wait. I'll get back at him when he least expects it! She leaned her head on his shoulder, laughing. "You'll be sorry."

After they sat out one dance, they were both eager to dance again. This time it was a rumba. They had such fun with it, they were hoping the band would play more Latin music. There wasn't anything Allen couldn't do, Jan was ready to burst the seams of her new red dress.

Quite a few of the girls danced with different guys, while Mandy sat there watching. At one point, Jan saw a tall, nice-looking guy ask Mandy to dance. Jan held her breath, hoping Mandy would accept and was blown away when she did!

As Jan and Allen danced around, she glimpsed the two of them talking to one another, moving slowly around the dance floor. When the dance ended, Jan watched them walk back to the table and was shocked to see him sit down beside her with a respectable distance between them as they continued to talk. He even got up and brought back cake and a drink. WOW! Jan was thrilled for Mandy!

"A penny for your thoughts, Pumpkin."

"I'm sorry, I've been watching Mandy and. . ."

"Is she doing something she's not supposed to do?"

"Oh heavens no. You see, I just found out that she's never dated and I saw this guy come over and ask her to dance, and now they're sitting together at the table visiting. I'm just so thrilled for her!"

"Oh, I see. He does look like a nice enough fellow, but I'll keep an eye on him just in case I have to rescue her."

"You certainly are my knight in shining armor."

"And I can dance too."

They continued to dance every dance until they needed a drink of water. They also decided to have a piece of cake while they sat down for a minute. Mandy introduced her new friend, Rob Shaw. He told them he was a new intern at the hospital.

Allen and Jan excused themselves when the last dance was announced. As they waltzed around the floor, Allen held Jan tightly in his arms while she laid her head on his shoulder. She was pleased to see Mandy and Rob dancing together as well. At the end of the dance, Allen kissed Jan tenderly, saying, "You are by far the best dance partner I've ever had."

Reluctantly they left and on the way home Jan asked, "How did you learn to dance so well?"

"My mother started me dancing when I was the age of two. She even put me into a stage show, dressed in a little white suit to dance for the audience."

"Did your folks love to dance?"

"Yes, they made quite a handsome couple at all of the local dances."

"How come I never knew this before?"

"Probably because you never asked. How did you learn to dance?"

"My father's a wonderful ballroom dancer. He taught me to dance when I was three by having me stand on top of his shoes in my stocking feet while he moved around to the music. I'm told that my folks took me to the World's Fair in San Francisco when I was about the same age and a band from Mexico was playing in an arena. They say I got up and danced in front of all the people and they gave me a standing ovation."

"See, I told you so!"

"Told me what?"

"That God was getting us ready to be together from the day we were born."

Allen walked her to the door. After kissing her, he said, "Thank you for giving me one of the most wonderful evenings of my life."

"Ditto. And now that I know you really can dance, I will most definitely marry you. Even though you're a pathological liar!" She closed the door behind her.

She could hear him laughing as he ran back to his car.

CHAPTER THIRTY THREE
WHAT IF HE TRIES SOMETHING?

Jan dreamed all night of dancing with Allen, but when she woke up she had to face a long day of study before Monday. In a little over six months she would be married, living in an apartment with Allen and studying for State Boards.

Mandy came down to Jan's room, and they went with a few others to eat breakfast. Most everyone was planning to stay at the dorm to study.

Kim asked, "Would you like to group study when we go back to the dorm?"

Nancy frowned and said "I'm not sure I feel like it, I think I'll just stay in my room."

Always the practical one, Mandy said, "Since we have some major finals next week, I think we should all agree to do it."

"We can do it first and it will be fun, to play our usual game?" Jan added.

Nancy groaned, "Okay, not more than an hour, okay?"

They agreed to play the game they invented in their freshman year when they had to memorize prefixes in medical terminology. They gathered together in their living room and took turns asking a question off the top of their head when they were sure of the answer. The first to answer correctly would be the one to ask the next question. They each took notes that would help them identify their individual weakness for further study. It was a good way to learn and prompted a lot of laughter and fun along with it.

When they finished, Mandy followed Jan into her room as was their custom, to study together. Mandy sat down and said, "I need to talk to you before we start studying."

"Sure, I wanted to talk to you also."

"Why don't you go first, Jan."

"Well, I was curious how you felt about Rob."

"You know, I really felt good around him. He was very nice both on and off the dance floor. It was easy to talk to him. But, Jan, I'm absolutely petrified of being alone with a man."

"Okay, I can understand why you feel that way, but I think you need to analyze where that fear is coming from. Why don't you ask yourself what image you have in your mind when you think of men."

"That's easy --- my rotten father."

"Do you think that all men are like your father?"

"I'm afraid they might become like him."

"Okay, let's look at this realistically. Do you think all of the men you have known since being in the nursing program might become like your father?"

"Well, not really all of them, but what if Rob is one of them?"

"Keep that in mind as we look at the whole picture. Imagine that you start dating him with the knowledge and insight you have acquired in these last few years. Do you think you might be smart enough to see some signs of a hidden agenda on his part?"

"Yes, I believe I could."

"Your knowledge is an important factor you have which I'm sure your mother couldn't possibly have had. She was barely wet behind the ears when she met your father. She had no education or basic insight into the character of a man. She was most likely in love with the idea of marriage and getting away from her responsibilities at home. He, on the other hand, just wanted a cook, a dishwasher and sex slave. Do you know if her parents approved of the marriage?"

"She told me that her mother really didn't like him, but her father was happy to get her out of the house because it meant one less mouth to feed."

"Now tell me how you felt when Rob first walked over and asked you to dance."

"A warm vibration took over my senses. Then when he asked me to dance, I felt light headed and extremely nervous. I told him I didn't know how to dance; then he said he couldn't dance very well either but was willing to give it a try if I would help him stand upright. I laughed and he just made me feel really comfortable."

"Do you mind if I try to analyze what you just told me?

"That's why I'm talking to Dr. Jan about it."

"When you say that you felt a warm vibration, that's exactly what I felt with Allen when he first talked to me at the college. I've met guys before and I've always felt everything from a sense of foreboding to mild interest, but I never felt what I felt with Allen. We are both convinced that God brought us together and that's probably why we're so completely drawn to one another. Now the other thing you mentioned was he made you feel comfortable. That was how I felt after Allen and I started to have a conversation together. Now tell me, have you thought about him since last night?"

"Jan, I can't stop thinking about him. I barely slept last night because he was so much in my thoughts."

"Did he ask if he could see you again?"

Mandy actually blushed as she answered, "He wants to take me to dinner tonight and I told him I would let him know. He gave me his phone number on this napkin," she said giggling, as she pulled it out of her pocket.

Jan looked at it and said, "Well what are you waiting for? Let's go down and call him immediately!"

"I'm scared my voice will be shaky. What do I say?"

"You keep it very simple. Just say you would love to go out to dinner tonight and that he should pick you up at the nurse's dorm. If he wants to talk, just tell him you have to get back to studying. Now let's get it over with so we can study." They ran downstairs, and Mandy ended up with a date for the evening.

* * *

In the late afternoon, Jan went with Mandy to her room and helped her pick out a dress for her date. Mandy took a shower, then Jan watched while Mandy put on her own makeup and combed out her hair. Some of the other girls got involved in picking out her accessories, mostly borrowed from others. When she was completely ready, they went down to the privacy of Jan's room. Mandy had told Jan she needed to talk to her alone before leaving.

When they were in Jan's room, Mandy turned to her and asked, "How should I react to him if he tries something?"

"First of all, I need to know what you personally consider 'something'?"

"Well, if he tries to hold me real close or kiss me, and especially if, well, you know what I mean?"

"Mandy, from what Allen and I observed of him, I really think he will be nothing but a gentleman. But to answer your question, if he tries to get fresh in any way, you just tell him that you are not that kind of girl. Holding hands should be acceptable, and a light hug is okay. I wouldn't shy away from a quick kiss, but anything more is too much, and just push him away. Does that sound comfortable to you?"

"Yes, I think I can handle that and hopefully survive the evening. I just wish I could get over this nervousness!"

"I can relate. I was the same with Allen at first. Just remember that he's probably a bundle of nerves also."

Jan watched her go out the door with Rob. He opened her car door. Jan could hardly wait for her to come home.

Jan went back to studying after a brief phone visit with Allen before he went to work.

* * *

Jan was getting cross eyed with drowsiness just as Mandy burst through Jan's door without bothering to knock. Jan jumped up, suddenly very much awake. She could tell from Mandy's expression that everything had gone well. Mandy was wearing a grin that didn't bother to stop at her earlobes.

Mandy talked like a magpie on caffeine. "Oh, Jan, he's so wonderful. He took me to a nice place downtown where the food was really good. He pulled my chair out for me and treated me like a queen. We talked about everything, and you will never believe this. He had an alcoholic father also. He's from a small town too, and he has no desire to ever see his father again. He was so polite and a little bit shy. All he did was hold my hand when we walked together. Jan, I've never felt like this before!"

"Mandy, I'm so happy for you. Did he ask if he could see you again?"

"Yes, right now he's working the night shift as part of his internship, so he's free in the early evenings except when his rotation comes up to be on call. Then he tells me that he pretty much grabs a nap in the hospital lounge. He asked if he could take me for a ride and picnic next Sunday afternoon."

"And?"

"I said yes of course!"

"Great. Now can we get some sleep? The alarm is going to go off way too soon."

"I don't think I can sleep, but I'll leave you alone so you can. Goodnight," she said as she hugged Jan, then closed the door behind her.

CHAPTER THIRTY FOUR
(1960)

A JOLT OF ELECTRICITY

Monday morning Jan was leaving her dorm room when Desirae called out, "Jan, wait for me." Des was slightly taller than Jan with the same colored hair and blue/green eyes.

Desirae said, "Hey girl, I think we're both going to the same rotation."

"Are you going to the psych ward?"

"You bet your sweet petunia I am."

Desirae was a lot of fun to be around, and Jan was happy to walk with her.

"Oh great, once you and I get in there, they'll probably never let us out." Jan laughed.

"That's okay with me. Just think of the fun we'll have. Say, while we walk over, tell me how Mandy's date went last night?"

"Great. She had a wonderful time, and he was a perfect gentlemen."

"Well, that's no fun! Just kidding. I'm so happy for Mandy. Let's face it; she isn't the type for men to knock down her door, right?"

"You have to give him credit for looking past her exterior to the beautiful person inside."

"You're so right. But I did notice, with makeup on, she really looked cute."

They walked through the hospital to a side elevator, and Jan excused herself to run up the stairs and meet her in front of the door to the Psychiatric Ward.

Des was waiting, "Here we are, ready or not. Jan, you first: age before beauty, you know."

Jan rang the bell for someone to come and unlock the door. As they waited, they could hear a loud female voice screaming obscenities at the top of her lungs. They looked at each other, and Jan said to Des, "Shall we put ourselves in reverse?"

The door opened and the colorful language blasted them out of their newly polished white nursing shoes. They could see a young woman in a hospital bed with wide leather wrist and ankle restraints attached to the bed frame. She was very thin, with black hair that looked as though it had been through a cement mixer. Dressed in filthy, torn clothing, the young woman had bloodshot eyes with pin-point pupils and looked as if she had come straight from the garbage dump.

Jan and Des stood there staring and wondered why she kept referring to her "mother" for help. The nurse that opened the door must have read their minds because she commented, "She isn't calling for her real mother. That's probably the last person she would want to see. That's a common term for their drug source on the street. She's been like this since she was admitted late last night. it'll be a few more hours, and then she'll crash for awhile. After that she'll be sicker than a dog!"

The nurse escorted Jan and Des into the nurses' station where they saw Miss Kingston waiting. Jan had long ago abandoned her fear of their instructor. Once she found out Miss Kingston was really quite human, she enjoyed being around her. Miss Kingston looked up as they walked in and said, "Welcome Miss Adler and Miss Winston. She gave Jan a slight smile and asked, "Was dancing with Allen everything you dreamed about?"

"Oh yes, and much better after I found out he had pulled a fast one on me."

"What on earth did he do, Miss Winston?"

"He told me he couldn't dance and even had me show him a few steps, then he took off on the dance floor like a professional!"

"Yes, we all noticed how well you danced together. He must be quite the tease."

"Oh yes, that he is."

"Okay, come along, students and I'll show you around."

As they toured, Jan and Des realized what a challenge they faced. It was easy to understand why this and emergency room were saved for their senior year. They were quite impressed with Miss Kingston's knowledge of psychiatric disorders and how easily she controlled some of the behavior problems they saw.

Miss Kingston confided, "This is one of my favorite places to work, with the exception of orthopedics-my first love."

They continued walking and Jan observed, "I'm surprised how large this part of the hospital is. It's uniquely laid out with so many different branches ending in separate areas. And so many locked doors."

"You're right Miss Winston, don't worry about the locked doors, you will each be given a master key."

Des said, "That's a relief."

"Just as a reminder, students, this will be your longest rotation, lasting three months." Miss Kingston said as they walked down a hall. "The first few weeks I will be here to guide you through, then you'll be on your own."

Just as they were about to round a corner, they ran into Kim. "Hi Miss Winston and Miss Adler. I've been here with Miss Newcastle for six weeks, and we're happy to have you join us, even if we won't see you real often. Miss Kingston really knows her stuff around here, so listen to her, okay? I have to run so I can assist with one of the patients going through a bad time following electric shock therapy."

As she ran off, Desirae asked Miss Kingston, "What did she mean, electric something?"

Miss Kingston replied, "Follow me down the hall and I'll show you."

They walked to another area, went through a locked door and entered a large empty room, with beds lined up in five rows. There were five beds in each row. Each bed was equipped with padded side rails, all empty at the moment. There was a machine at the end of each row with a headband device dangling with wires that connected to a box apparatus containing a display of dials, buttons and knobs. The apparatus looked like a prop for a Frankenstein movie. There was a container of padded tongue blades on top of the machine, which Jan remembered making in Central Supply during her two week rotation there.

Jan looked around, and turned to Miss Kingston, asking, "What goes on in here?"

"This is where we treat those patients who don't respond to psychotherapy and/or medications. They are usually suffering from severe schizophrenia, depression, anxiety or dissociative disorders. It is called electroshock therapy."

"You mean they're jolted with electricity?"

"Yes, Miss Winston. It has proven to be a very successful treatment in these cases."

Then Jan made the biggest faux pas of her nursing career right in front of Miss Kingston.

CHAPTER THIRTY FIVE
FOOT IN MOUTH DISEASE

"But, Miss Kingston, electric shock could kill a person!"

"Miss Winston, step into the hall immediately!"

Miss Kingston was visibly angry as they stepped out the door and it wasn't until then, that Jan noticed some patients had been brought to the other end of the room. She knew she was in really big trouble.

Jan faced Miss Kingston, and all of the fear she felt in her first year swept over her like Niagara Falls. Miss Kingston looked like she was about to throw Jan over those falls handcuffed inside an old, smelly trunk.

"Miss Winston, what is one of the first principles you were taught about conversations around patients?"

"Never to talk about their condition or anything that would frighten them. And I did just that, didn't I?"

"Miss Winston, what you just did was inexcusable as a senior nearing the end of her training. I'm very tempted to give you an immediate leave of absence to ponder what you've just done and force you to make up this rotation in the summer! That would automatically extend your time for state boards to January of 1961. I need to ponder this action and talk to Mrs. Caspar before making a final decision. Before doing so, I need to ask you one question. Since your back was facing the area of the room that the patients had entered, were you aware they were present?"

"Absolutely not! But even then, I should have looked around before saying anything to make sure we were still alone in the room. I'm so sorry I made such a horrible mistake!"

"Alright, for now that will do. However, I must consider this, and I will get back to you. Now, please come back into the room so you can observe the procedure with Miss Adler."

They walked back in. Des and Jan exchanged knowing glances before watching the procedure. Nothing could have prepared them for what followed. Most of the patients were medicated prior to the procedure. Some still fought against it, but their efforts were useless against the strength of the orderlies. As soon as the band was placed around his or her forehead, the doctor started the electric shock. Quickly the nurse would place the padded tongue blade between his or her teeth and stand by the bed to keep watch over the individual as the shock to their brain developed into a full blown grand mal seizure.

Jan was in shock herself. *I can't believe what I'm seeing. I've seen many seizures from epilepsy, but this is a "man made" seizure. I can't believe they have purposely inflicted such torture on a human being!* Once the seizure ended, the individual fell into a deep sleep. Jan and Des sighed with relief.

Miss Kingston, spoke, "They will be sleeping for a couple of hours, so we'll resume our tour."

They turned and walked down to the end of the hall where the day room was located. She turned to the students. "I'm going to let you nurses walk around and see if you can engage in some conversations or one on one interaction. I'll be within earshot if you have a question or problem." She turned around and left them standing there.

By then, Jan's feelings tumbled in an internal mixer. She wanted little to do with mingling with a bunch of crazies. Feeling totally inadequate, she looked around the room and settled on a woman sitting in a chair with her right arm held over her head. Her other arm hugged her waist and she stared straight ahead, not moving a muscle. Jan approached her and said, "Hi, I'm Miss Winston, are you enjoying being in the day room?" The women didn't move a muscle. "Can you tell me your name?" Complete silence. "Would you like to take a walk with me?" Still nothing. The women continued to stare into outer space. "I'll visit with you again soon."

Jan recognized the patient's behavior. Curious to see if she was correct, Jan found her way back to the nurses' station and asked, "Could I see the chart of the catatonic female patient in the day room?"

"So, the pretty little student nurse is diagnosing patients now?" A male voice said from behind the desk. "Miss Kingston, what are you teaching these nurses lately?"

Jan felt the heat rising to her face. *What have I done; am I in more trouble?*

"Dr. Whooly, Miss Winston is one of our best students and remembers what she's been taught." Miss Kingston said, coming to Jan's defense.

"Whoa, I was teasing you, Miss Kingston and her diagnosis dovetails quite nicely with mine. It just so happens she's absolutely right." He stood up from the desk, handing Jan a chart as he asked, "And does the best student in class wish to take a seat?"

"I'm not allowed to when a doctor is present, but thank you for the chart."

He put out his other hand to take hers. "You are more than welcome to sit beside me, Miss Winston. I'm the chief psychopath here, and I welcome you to our nutty ward."

Jan couldn't help but laugh as he smiled at her. She was struck by his piercing blue eyes. She judged him to be in his mid thirties, with a receding hairline that pushed back his light brown hair.

Miss Kingston spoke up. "Miss Winston, you're welcome to take a seat."

"It's really all right?"

"Yes, just ignore him. He's only a psychiatrist. He doesn't count."

Dr. Whooly chuckled. "Oh, good one, Miss Kingston, payback time, I see."

"I'm never one to miss an opportunity."

I think I'm going to enjoy it here and Miss Kingston is back to her good old self.

Jan read the patient's history and learned her name was Ruby; then returned to the day room. She stopped to talk to a couple of patients working on a puzzle. "Hi, my name is Miss Winston. Can you tell me your names?"

One man answered, "I'm Tom and He's Jerry," He laughed hysterically.

Jerry said in an angry tone, "Knock it off ,Tom. If you keep laughing, I'll tear the puzzle apart!"

"Tear the puzzle, tear the puzzle, tear the puzzle, tear the puzzle, tear the puzzle, tear the puzzle, tear the puzzle, . . ."

"Tom, shut up! You sound like you're crazy!" said Jerry as he got up and stomped back to his room.

Jan asked Tom, "May I work the puzzle with you?"

"Miss Winston work the puzzle, work the puzzle, work the puzzle, work the puzzle, work the puzzle, work the puzzle, . . ."

"Tom, that's enough. Now stop." Miss Kingston said from behind Jan.

Jan added a few pieces, then stood to look around. Des was in a conversation with a patient in the corner, so she ventured over to a teenager sitting alone on a couch. "Hi, I'm Miss Winston. Can you tell me your name?"

In a very small voice she answered, "Suzy."

"I like that name. How old are you, Suzy?"

"I'm 16 and they put me in here with a bunch of crazy people."

"Well, I'm here, and I'm not crazy."

"What are you then?"

"I'm a student nurse."

"Is that why you're dressed in that funny costume?"

"This is my uniform."

"What are those stripes on your sleeve? Are you a sergeant?"

"It means I'm a senior and I'm going to graduate in a few months. Then I can work as a regular nurse."

"Is it fun being a nurse?"

"Most of the time it is."

She leaned in real close, glancing around to make sure no one could hear her, "You know Miss Winston, I'm here by mistake. My parents made them take me by telling a bunch of lies about me. Maybe you can help me get out of here then I can run away."

"Suzy, I can't do that because I don't have a key."

"Didn't they give you a key?"

"No."

"Oh!" With that Suzy got up and walked out of the day room.

Again, Jan went back to the nurses' station to look at charts. Des was there and reported that her own conversation with Suzy was much the same.

Des handed her Suzy's chart and said, "You will find this most interesting."

As Jan read, she was fascinated. Suzy had been admitted in a delusional state of paranoid schizophrenia. Her parents stated she had taken herself off medication and was experiencing periods of severe psychoses. The most recent episode involved rubbing herself all over her naked body with her own feces, stating she was cleansing herself of evil spirits. When her parents tried to coax her into the shower, she ran into the kitchen and threatened them with a large butcher knife. The father called the police and they subdued her, then brought her to the hospital. Her behavior was much better controlled with medication.

On the way out, Miss Kingston put a master key in each of their hands and said it was best to pin it inside their blue uniform pocket that would be covered by their white apron. Jan went to lunch wondering how long she would have to wait for Miss Kingston's decision. It lay heavy on her mind.

CHAPTER THIRTY SIX
A WOLF IN PASTOR'S CLOTHING

"I went to see a preacher this morning" said Allen, as he drove Jan to her afternoon classes. "He seemed nice enough, but he asked me some very personal questions, making me feel uncomfortable."

"Like what kind of questions?"

"I'd rather not say, Pumpkin; he did ask me to bring you to church this Sunday. Afterward he wants to talk to you alone."

"Why can't we talk to him together?"

"Honey, if I knew, I'd tell you, but he must have his reasons."

"Okay, fine, we'll go Sunday; but he better be careful what he asks me."

"Jan, keep in mind, he's the only minister that agreed to marry us without our being members of his congregation."

"Did you really check all of the different churches, and they all said no?"

"Well, in a way. They were hesitant or asked us to join their congregation."

"Wow, I had no idea they're so strict."

"Well, if we start going every Sunday between now and when we get married, they would probably do it."

"We don't have time to do that. See you later," said Jan as Allen let her off near her class.

* * *

Sunday they drove to church, found an empty pew and sat down. Everyone was very quiet, but many were openly turning around in their seats to check them out. The congregation started by singing a familiar hymn and Jan could hear Allen singing above the others. They held hands and enjoyed hearing the choir sing a special gospel number during the service. They watched as the preacher strolled to the pulpit. Jan nearly jumped out of her dress when he slammed the Bible down and with a roaring voice said, "According to this book," slamming it again, "you are all sinners! Each and every one of you! You have come today to redeem your souls, and tomorrow you will envy your neighbor. You will lust after your brother's wife. You will tell a lie. You will take from the poor by spending money on fancy clothes!"

At this point Jan wanted to slink out of there and never come back. Remembering what Allen had told her, she endured the rest of his degrading sermon in agony. There was another enjoyable song from the choir, some passages read from the Bible, and after a closing hymn, they made their way to his office while people stared as if they were covered in green hair.

The preacher walked up, shook Allen's hand and said, "Allen, please wait outside while Janet and I visit inside my office." He opened the door. "Janet, please have a seat inside," he said, pointing to a chair. Instead of sitting behind his desk, he pulled up a second chair between Jan and the door, facing her. His penetrating brown eyes glittered and his face lit up with a smile that revealed very large teeth. Jan could smell his offensive breath, and shivered as if she were cold.

In a soft voice he asked, "Janet, I understand you would like me to officiate at your wedding?"

"Correct."

"To do so, I feel it is very important for me to get to know you better, would you agree?"

"I suppose so." *Where's he going with this?*

He reached for her hand, and she drew it back. *It's bad enough you have to sit so close, I'm not letting you touch me, you repulsive, smelly man.*

"I'm sorry. Do I offend you?"

"I just don't feel comfortable with you holding my hand."

"My goodness, are you afraid of men?"

"No, of course not."

"You do realize intimacy is a part of the marriage covenant. Maybe you need some coaching to help you relax around a man." he said, as he placed his hand on her knee.

"I don't think it's necessary for you to touch me and I do not like where this conversation is going!"

"Now Janet, relax. I'm just trying to be friendly. I need to ask you some questions. Are you all right with that?"

"It depends on the questions." She swiveled her knees away from his groping hand.

"I understand. Tell me your feelings about your future husband."

"I'm very much in love with him."

"Do you feel comfortable when he kisses you?"

"Of course."

With a crooked smile he asked, "Has he touched you anywhere that aroused new feelings in you?"

"No, and I don't like your insinuations. I think I'm ready to leave!"

He stood up in front of her, blocking her way. "Now Janet, I mean you no harm." He placed his hands on her shoulders, "I'm acting under the authority of God, and I need to know a lot more about you. I have to ask these questions before I can solemnize your marriage. Do you understand?" His hand brushed against her breast as she pushed him away.

"I completely understand, and I don't want to talk to you anymore." She said through gritted teeth. Jan tried to go around him as he thrust a paper in front of her and put his hand out to make her sit down.

He moved dangerously close to her, "Please, at least take time to answer these questions so I can consider performing your ceremony."

Jan grabbed the form, glanced at the questions and felt such a revulsion that she threw the paper down. She stood and pushed past him with a sense of urgency. The door was locked. "You locked this door on purpose?"

"Yes, but I can explain."

"Don't waste your breath," Jan said between clenched teeth. "Unlock this door immediately, or I'll scream RAPE!"

"Now, now, calm down, Missy." He took the key from his pocket and unlocked the door.

She rushed out to Allen, grabbed his hand and pulled him down the hall to escape.

In the safety of the car, she spoke in an angry voice, "Allen, he's a despicable man! Tell me where he sat when you went to his office to talk to him."

"Behind his desk. Why?"

Jan told Allen the whole story, ending with, "He locked the door, put his chair close to me, then he put his hand on my knee and demanded I fill out a form."

"He what?"

"He locked the door and I . . ."

Allen was out of the car before Jan could think of what he might do. She got out, running behind. "Allen, don't go in there. Just leave it be!"

Allen didn't acknowledge Jan's plea as he tore back into the church with Jan on his heels.

"Open this door, you freak!" He tried the locked door, then kicked it as a few choice words flew out of his mouth.

"Allen, please, let's just go!" People stared at them like their hair had turned to spikes of marble.

Allen stood in the hall, with his hands to his sides, fists clenched. Jan stepped up and took his hand, pulling him down the hall like a disobedient child.

They got into the car and just sat there.

"Allen, do you want me to drive?"

"No, I'm sorry. It's a good thing his door was locked. I probably would have massacred the guy. He started the engine and slowly left the parking lot. "What do we do now? No church and no minister and we have a wedding in a few months."

As they drove slowly down the street, Jan saw other churches along the way. "Did you check that one?" Each time he said "Yes, have to be a member," or whatever. They came upon another and another, and Jan kept asking. They drove on in silence for awhile, and as they passed a side street, Jan spotted a church down the street.

"Allen, did you stop at the one down the street we just passed?"

"Where? What?"

"Go around the corner up here and drive around to see what it looks like."

As they approached, they saw a stately brick building landscaped with lawn, flower beds and green shrubs. Allen hesitantly pulled into the parking lot filled with cars.

"Jan, do you think we should go in? It's afternoon, but it looks like they're having services right now."

"Are you calmed down enough to be on your best behavior?"

"Yes, I'm okay. Let's just peek inside."

They went up the steps, cracked open the door and heard someone talking. There was a lobby with couches and chairs, but the doors to the chapel were closed, and a female voice was talking about the importance of showing love to everyone. They exchanged glances as they felt a remarkable difference from the horror of the morning. They sat on the couch and listened. A man with an incredible voice sang a beautiful song about the Savior's love. Then they heard a man talking about the greatest commandment in Matthew 22. They held hands and sat listening, feeling a little bit like eavesdroppers.

An organ played as the congregation sang "God be with you 'til we meet again." The doors opened, and they felt extremely conspicuous sitting on the couch as people poured out of the chapel, smiling and talking among themselves. Some came over to shake their hands. One such gentleman approached and asked, "May I help you find someone?"

"Yes, we'd like to talk to your minister."

"That would be me. My name is Scott Conklin. And yours?"

"I'm Allen Morris, and this is my fiancée Janet Winston. But before we waste your time, do you require couples to be members of your church to marry them?"

"Why don't we go down to my office and I'll explain our requirements."

Allen and Jan followed him down the hall and entered an office with the picture of Jesus Christ on the wall behind his desk. He pulled up a couple of chairs for them and said, "When do you intend to get married?"

"If possible, the second Saturday in June."

"Okay, the first thing I have to check is whether the building is already scheduled for that particular Saturday." He reached for a book from the corner of his desk, flipping the pages. Oh, I was afraid of this. We have a special meeting for our ladies on that date. Ah, but the following Saturday is free. Let's talk a bit before we schedule it."

"You mean you will marry us here without us being members of your church?"

"Yes, but I do need to ask a few questions first."

Oh, great. Here we go again. I'm tempted to get up and walk out right now. Jan half rose to push her chair back, when Allen spoke.

"What kinds of questions?"

"To be married in our chapel, which we consider sacred, I need to ask if you're living certain standards."

"What kind of standards?"

"Well, for example, we don't allow any liquor or smoking in or around our building. And for you to be married in our chapel, you need to have remained chaste."

Jan was baffled as she asked, "What does chaste mean?"

Allen laughed, "No sex before marriage."

"Oh," Jan said as she felt the heat rise to her cheeks. "We've done that. I mean we haven't done that! I mean we are what you said. I'm so embarrassed!"

Both men were laughing, as Jan felt like a fumbling idiot.

"Janet, has Allen treated you in a respectable manner at all times?"

Janet couldn't help snickering a bit as she answered, "Yes, except when he lies about not knowing how to dance."

Allen spoke up, "That wasn't lying, that was teasing."

Jan laughed, "And I was just teasing to get back at you."

The minister gave a hearty laugh and said, "Sounds like you two have a healthy relationship. How long have you been dating?"

Allen answered, "Too long. Over two years."

"Okay, give me your names again, I'm putting it on the calendar. And if you desire, your reception can be in our hall."

"Oh, ah, how much do you charge for everything?" Allen asked.

"There's no charge."

"Well, what do you charge for the marriage ceremony?"

"Nothing."

Allen and Jan looked at each other in disbelief.

"One more thing, we need to know how many people you expect and when you want to decorate, etc. And let me write down the address for your invitations. There you go."

As they started to leave he said, "Oh, I almost forgot, I need a couple of phone numbers to reach you if I think of something else."

After exchanging phone numbers, they shook hands and walked out in a stupor.

They got in the car and Jan said, "What just happened?"

"I think our guardian angels have struck again!"

CHAPTER THIRTY SEVEN
THE PUNISHMENT

After the first couple of weeks Jan and Desirae enjoyed working the psych ward. They watched as the woman they had originally seen in those leather restraints began her long road back to sobriety. She had been deathly sick for almost two weeks, now she had transitioned to a manipulating, angry monster.

Jan observed her sitting in the middle of the floor in the day room. She had positioned herself so people would have to step over or around her to get to the games. *Did she want attention or what?* Jan went up to her and asked, "Rita, why are you sitting in the middle of the floor?"

"'Cause I can sit wherever I well please, and what's it to you anyway?"

"Just curious," Jan said as she walked away and sat on the couch.

Rita wasn't getting much attention, so she walked over next to Jan. "Why do you wear such a stupid outfit?"

"This is my uniform and we're required to wear it."

"Nobody could tell me what to wear. I'd tell 'em to shove it up their rosy red . .!"

"Okay, okay, that's fine for you, but I don't mind it a bit."

"You're sure a little tiny thing. A good wind would blow you away. Hey, you want to have a cigarette with me?"

"I don't smoke, but I don't mind if you do."

"Hey, you're all right. What's your name?"

"Miss Winston."

"It sure would be nice if you'd walk around outside with me while I smoke."

"That would be nice, but I'm not allowed to take anyone outside. You can smoke in the day room."

"I said I wanted to go outside!" The language used would have better served had it stuck in her throat.

Suddenly Rita decided to continue her temper tantrum in the day room. Everything not nailed down Rita hurled into the next century, scattering several screaming, angry patients from one side of the room to another. Puzzle pieces paraded into orbit; anything she could break shattered to pieces; she overturned every piece of furniture before four strong orderlies were able to subdue her. *This must be what it feels like to be in the middle of a war zone, dodging debris and heavy artillery.*

The orderlies took her to an area that was used for out-of-control substance abuse patients. Jan had never seen it in use, so she tagged along. It was a large room with what looked like three extra large bath tubs standing on end. Across from them, a fire hose dripping ice cold water stood ready for action. The orderlies placed her in the middle of one of these "tubs" and fastened her wrists in restraints after stripping her down to just her underwear. One of the orderlies went to the fire hose and turned the freezing water on her, forcing her body against the back of the tub. She screamed in agony. Even though Jan had no great feelings for Rita, she felt as though her heart would break in two! *How can they do this? This is even more torture than electroshock therapy.* After what seemed like a very long time, he eased the temperature up to warm, then stopped it.

Rita whimpered, "I'm freezing, help me before I die." She shivered as if she'd been standing in the icy wind of the north pole. Janet assisted the other nurses with towels to wipe her off, wrapped her in a warm blanket and escorted Rita to her room. She curled her shaking body into a ball under the covers.

Dr. Whooly came in and sat on the edge of the bed and talked softly to Rita. "I'm sorry you had to go through this Rita. Your behavior in the day room was not acceptable. Can you tell me why you felt so angry?"

"That cutesy little nurse wouldn't take me outside to have a cigarette!" she said, pointing at Jan.

"Was she mean to you?"

"No."

"What did she say to you?"

"She's not allowed to take me out."

"And was she mean to you?"

"No, damn it. I already told you she wasn't!"

"Then there must have been something else making you angry enough to demolish the day room. Can you dig down deep inside and think of something that has made you angry for a very long time?"

"I want my mother!"

"Are you referring to your street mother?"

"Yeah, I don't like the way you're prying into my head. I need to get out of this place!" She tried to sit up.

Dr. Whooly purposely blocked her from sitting. "Rita, I want you to go back in time and tell me when you began to feel so angry."

"You're an idiot. Why should I go back to remembering being hated and neglected by my parents? Why did they lock me in my room for days? Why did they ignore my pleas to use the bathroom until I'd shit my pants? Why? Please find my mother. NOW PLEASE!"

Just then the nurse came in to give her a tranquilizing injection, and as she was leaving, she gestured to Jan to follow her out. "Miss Winston, Miss Kingston wants to talk to you."

Her instructor's name brought back the realization that she was still waiting for the guillotine to drop regarding her previous mistake with a patient. It had been over a month. She walked to the nurses' station and greeted Miss Kingston.

"Miss Winston, since it's almost time for lunch, please follow me to my office." Jan silently followed her out of the psych unit and into the main hospital to her office.

"Please have a seat," Miss Kingston said as she made herself comfortable behind her desk. "Miss Winston, I apologize for taking so long to get back to you regarding your suspension." Jan's heart jumped to the back of her throat.

Consumed by weakness, Jan feebly answered, "It's all right, Miss Kingston."

"I have talked the matter over with Mrs. Caspar, and we are in agreement. Because of your outstanding behavior in the past and what I have observed in the last month, we will waive suspension. However, because this comes under the subject of 'Professional Ethics' and having completed that course last semester we are removing the 'A' you received and replacing it with a 'D'"

Jan's heart took a nosedive into a deep pit of despair. She had worked so hard to maintain a high grade point average and this would be on her record forever. It would have felt better to be suspended.

"Is that your final decision?"

"Yes, Miss Winston. The change has already been made. You're excused."

"Thank you, Miss Kingston."

As Jan walked the dorm, she could feel every fiber of her being twisted into knots. She felt physically ill and not sure if she could face anyone right now. She saw Allen waiting at the car, gave him a limp wave before she changed her clothes for college. The minute he hugged her she began to cry and pour her heart out to him. He talked to her for a long time before class and she was feeling much better by the time he left her.

* * *

On the way home, Allen said "I've been thinking, since our wedding is only a few months away, we should start looking for an apartment."

"Doesn't it seem a little early for us to be looking?"

"Well, yes, except I'm already renting a room with a bath, and that costs me $50 a month, plus I have the expense of eating out and a couple of dollars a day adds up. Of course, sometimes I buy a loaf of bread and some bologna for about 35 cents and those last me quite a few meals. Then when I take my fiancée out, she orders prime rib and I'm broke for a couple more weeks."

"Wait a minute, I eat a lot of hot dogs when I go out with you."

"Oh yeah, I forgot. All kidding aside, I've been looking in the ads and there's a lot of places available centrally located between the University and Watkins Medical Center. And not very far from the gas station. Do you want me to start looking? If I like a few, I can take you over to see them?"

"Okay, but I'm very particular, you know."

"Oh, how well I know. It took me a long time to convince you to fall in love with me."

"Right, all of two minutes after our eyes locked together."

"Two minutes can seem like forever."

They laughed, and he left her off at the dorm so he could go to work.

CHAPTER THIRTY EIGHT
THE WRATH OF RITA

When Jan told Mandy and the other students about her punishment, they wanted to go and talk to Mrs. Caspar. Jan explained that even if they did, it was too late to change anything; the indelible ink was signed on the dotted line, and she would have to live with her error in judgment the rest of her life.

The next morning Jan entered a ward and saw a female patient in her sixties coming down the hall. The patient called herself "Miss Judy" and would walk around the hall with her right index finger pushing into the center of her back just below her waistline; giving the impression she was pushing herself around the hall. "Hello, Miss Judy. How are you today?"

Standing less than five-feet tall, with gray hair cut short and pale blue eyes, she stopped in front of Jan and place her feet apart as if she were about to pitch a baseball. She placed her left hand on her hip, displayed a crocked smile that revealed yellow teeth and answered in a squeaky voice while elongating each word saying, "Yeess, I'mmm fiine. Yeess, I'mmm Missss Juudy. Yeess, I liike to waallkk. You're very pretty."

Before more could be said, she turned and started pacing again. Judy had been hospitalized in mental institutions all her life and had never known anything different. Harmless in every way, she would have perished in the real world without someone to take care of her.

On the same ward, Jan kept a watchful eye on "Mattie." She stood over six-feet tall and was about 40 pounds overweight. Her short brown hair was styled in a pageboy and Mattie's hazel eyes were circled with red rims. The patient walked with a slight limp, curling her upper back forward, and stared at people, slowly revealing her smile of sharp pointed teeth. She reminded Jan of the Hunchback of Notre Dame. Jan had been told she would come up behind some of the nurses and grab them around their shoulders and squeeze. Mattie was also a thief. She often took linens off other beds and towels from the bathrooms, then hid them under her mattress. Jan could just imagine Mattie grabbing her and stuffing her like a rag doll under her mattress to play with later. Jan successfully avoided making any close contact with her, always mindful of her back.

Jan often returned to Rita's ward so she could measure her progress. One day she arrived while Rita was back in the "water tank" after beating up another patient when he told her to move out of the way. Jan watched the treatment again and followed Dr. Whooly to Rita's room. He didn't stay as long this time so Jan followed him to the nurses' station to ask some questions. When she walked in, Jan heard him say, "I'm going to try her on some electroshock therapy and see if I can get her to the point where I'll be able to break through to her anger."

Jan knew he was not one to use this therapy indiscriminately, so she approached him. "Hi Dr. Whooly. May I sit down and ask some questions?"

"Only if you know the answers so you can tell me."

Jan laughed. "Now I was being serious."

"Well, so was I!"

"Dr. Whooly, I really have some important questions to ask. Are you ready?"

"Absolutely, Miss Winston. What would you like to know?"

"Does electroshock therapy leave any permanent damage to the patient's brain?"

"Good question. We know it does cause changes to occur in the brain resulting in a higher level of manageability in the patient. It's not known at this time if there is any permanent damage, but let me point out that it is by far a better treatment than a partial or complete frontal lobectomy."

"Dr. Whooly, 'ectomy' means surgical removal. Would you elaborate?

"Yes, we remove part or all of the frontal lobe in the brain on patients who don't respond to any other form of treatment. Lobectomy is used as a very last resort and only when patients are an extreme danger to themselves or others."

"They just take out part of the brain and throw it away?"

"Yes, Miss Winston. Come with me and I'll take you to the ward where we care for these patients. As you observe, keep in mind these people were violent towards themselves and others. No medication or other method of treatment controlled them except this."

He unlocked a door and walked in with Jan. Men and women paced up and down the hall. He stopped one of them and she looked at him with eyes devoid of any emotion, then looked past him into space. He asked her, "How are you today?" There was no acknowledgment and he moved aside so she could continue her walk.

Jan felt sick as she quietly said, "She's no longer a person."

"Sadly, you're right. But the alternative would be far sadder to watch. And much more frightening."

In the day room a man was walking around picking up papers and setting them back down. Then he picked up magazines and put them back down. All the while he talked to himself in gibberish. Another was staring out the window almost in a catatonic state.

Jan turned to Dr. Whooly and asked, "Have all these patients had a lobectomy?"

"Pretty much."

"Well, if I ever have to go through that, will you make sure I'm doing the magazines and papers. At least I would be busy."

"Miss Winston, I wouldn't lose any sleep over it."

"Thanks for showing me around. Can we go back to the more exciting ward now?"

"Sure."

When they returned to the ward, Jan walked down the hall to find Rita. She was sitting on her bed, and Jan walked in greeting her. "Hi, Rita. Do you mind if I sit down and visit for awhile?"

"If I say no, you'll do it anyway, right?"

"No, if you don't want me here, I'll leave." Jan turned to step out.

"Fine, stay if you want."

"Do you feel like talking?"

Rita was angry. "You're all the same. Everyone wants me to talk. Well, maybe I don't want to!"

"No problem. Do you want to walk down to the day . . . . " Jan never saw it coming. She was suddenly flying across the room, sliding down the wall, with Rita on top of her as everything went dark.

She woke up on a gurney moving fast down the hall with Dr. Whooly on one side, an orderly and Des on the other. Jan was overcome by extreme pain in her nose, cheeks and forehead. "What happened to me?"

"Just lay quiet, Miss Winston. Rita decided to take her frustrations out on your face, but you'll be fine. We're on our way to emergency so they can take care of you." Dr. Whooly tried to reassure her.

"Is Rita okay?"

"She's in our quiet room right now, and she's scheduled for electroshock this afternoon."

Wish I were in the quiet room right about now, padded walls, no furniture, soft cushy floor. I could just curl into a ball and hide in the corner. Then I could make believe this never happened to me.

As they arrived in the emergency room, Miss Kingston was there to greet her. X-ray revealed a fractured nose. They packed it, taped it and Des escorted her back to the dorm to rest with an ice pack. She took a couple of aspirin and laid on her bed with the ice.

She was suddenly startled awake with Mandy leaning over her, "Jan Winston, what on earth happened to you?"

"I was trampled by a herd of wild cattle." she whispered with a nasal voice.

"Jan, this isn't funny, tell me what happened."

"I had a small confrontation with a patient in the psych ward."

"Oh my gosh, my next rotation will be there. Maybe I shouldn't go!"

"Hey, you're big enough to take care of yourself. Where were you when I needed protecting?"

"I would have taken care of him for sure."

"Mandy, it wasn't a 'he', it was a 'her'."

"Oh, you are a ninety-five pound weakling, aren't you?"

"Mandy, would you look out the window and see if Allen's waiting for me?"

Mandy walked over and said, "He's there. Are you going to your college classes?"

"Of course."

"Okay, I'll run and warn him. He's going to have a hemorrhage when he sees you!"

Mandy ran out her door, and Jan got up slowly, feeling dizzy while sitting on the edge of the bed. She was determined to go to school even though she knew it wasn't the smartest thing to do. She looked in the mirror to comb her hair and almost fainted. Both of her eyes were swollen and turning a variety of colors from pink to red to purple. Her hair looked like someone had poured a bucket of water over her, and blood was caked around the packing and her lips. She went to the bathroom and cleaned up the best she could, picked up her books and gingerly walked down the steps.

Allen was standing in the doorway with Mandy. As she came into view, he gazed at her like she was a freak in a circus side show "Oh, no, I don't believe it!"

"I don't either."

"Sweetheart, you shouldn't be going anywhere."

"I'm not going to miss class and jeopardize my grades any more than they already are."

Allen turned to Mandy, "I guess there's no arguing with her. Do you have the same class as Jan?"

"I sure do and I'll take good care of her."

"Thanks, Mandy; okay, let me walk you to the car, Pumpkin."

By the time Allen let Janet off at the dorm following classes, she felt like a scuba diver who had collided head-on with a submarine. Jan's eyes were nearly swollen shut, her head felt like it would explode any minute. The inability to breath took her back to flashbacks of those last minutes in the elevator. When she stepped inside, Miss Kingston surprised her by greeting her at the door.

"Hello, Miss Winston, I came to see how you're feeling."

"Not too good at the moment."

"You didn't have to go to school, you know. I admire your courage, but it wasn't necessary. You would have been better off resting with an ice pack."

"I know that now and I'll sleep with an ice pack tonight."

"Miss Winston, tomorrow is Thursday. I'm excusing you from the ward tomorrow and Friday morning, and I'll allow you to make the decision whether to attend classes or not."

"Thank you, Miss Kingston."

She could barely drag herself up the stairs where Mandy was waiting with an ice pack.

"Okay, my foolish friend, I've volunteered to be your private duty nurse tonight. You know, if you keep up this kind of radical behavior, Allen and I will divorce you!"

"Mandy, I need to ask you a question. How are you and Rob getting along?"

"Oh, you sure know how to avoid my wrath, switching my train of thought to Rob. We're doing just fine. I haven't seen a lot of him lately because he's been on call non-stop at the hospital. He leaves me little notes where I'm working right now and calls me when he gets a break."

"Oh good. Have you told him about the wedding?"

"Yes and he's already received permission to have that weekend off."

"Good. Give me the ice pack, I think I need to take a nap now."

CHAPTER THIRTY NINE
CINDY, THAT'S RAPE

By Monday the swelling in Jan's face was down. With the packing removed, she looked almost human again with the exception of her multi-colored eyes and nose.

Dr. Whooly greeted her as she walked in. "Miss Winston, you are a sight for sore nose, I mean eyes. How are you feeling, young lady?"

"I'm much better, thank you, but I do have a question."

"Shoot."

"I had no indication this was coming when I sat down with Rita. Is there something I could have done to prevent it?"

"I think you know by now, psych patients are unpredictable. Rita has been treading thin water managing her anger for some time now. For that very reason, I had ordered electroshock therapy that very afternoon. I believe you were in the wrong place at the wrong time and she was just looking for a candidate for her rage."

"How is she now?"

"Let's go visit her, and you can see for yourself."

"As long as you're with me, I'll go."

They walked down the hall together. When Jan saw Rita, she was sitting on her bed reading a book-something she'd never seen her do before."

Rita looked up, set her book aside and said, "Hello, Dr. Whooly. As she glanced at Jan, she took in a quick breath and asked, "What happened to your face?"

"I ran into a bus."

Dr. Whooly sat down next to Rita. "Actually, Rita, you did that to Miss Winston last week."

"I would never do something like that!"

"Rita, remember how we've been talking about some of the things that happened to you in your childhood?"

"Yes"

"And how you had taken all of your anger and stuffed it deep down inside of you?"

"Yes"

"Well, before you allowed yourself to talk about it, you were taking your anger out on other people and things. Do you remember?"

"Oh, Miss Winston, did I really do that to you?"

"Yes, Rita, you did."

"I'm so sorry."

Dr. Whooly spoke up. "You are both going through a healing process at this time and Rita you have made great strides on your road to recovery. I'm real proud of you."

He got up to leave and as they walked down the hall, Dr. Whooly commented, "Does the change in her behavior surprise you?"

"It astounds me!"

"Does it give you a new perspective of electroshock therapy?"

"Yes, most certainly."

Miss Kingston greeted Jan at the nurses' station and told her she would be assisting with the electroshock treatments for this week. Even though it was hard for Jan to watch, she could now see the benefit of the treatments. But she still thought the cold water punishment was inhumane. She enjoyed the rest of her rotation there, and by the time it was over, her nose was almost back to normal with just a hint of pale yellow around her eyes. Her friends teased that she was lucky she didn't end up with a cauliflower nose.

* * *

One afternoon in nursing class, Miss Kingston made an announcement. "Students, graduation is looming closer, and it is time to elect a class valedictorian. Only our top scholastic students are eligible. I'm handing out papers with four names on them, and you are to vote for the one you wish to represent you at your graduation."

Jan had a sinking feeling; her previous punishment would disqualify her. At the same time she felt relief knowing her panic would return if she had to give a speech in front of a huge crowd. She received her piece of paper and saw Mandy's name at the top; the end was her own name. She was shocked, but it didn't matter; she was voting for Mandy.

They folded and handed in the papers. Miss Kingston gave them to Mrs. Jacob to tally the votes. After class, they took a short break, then Miss Kingston stood with a paper in her hand.

"Ladies, I have the results of your votes. I might add, this includes the votes of your instructors as well. Your valedictorian for the Watkins Medical Center's 1960 nursing graduating class is, by unanimous vote, Miss Janet Winston!"

The sudden clapping stunned Jan. She wanted to melt and disappear. Jan was well aware she could say or do nothing to change this. Common sense reminded her, she needed to face her demons. Janet stood up and said, "Thank you. I'm sincerely honored."

Invitations for her graduation and wedding had been prepared by her mom to be mailed. The wedding dress was purchased, showers had been given and Allen was now living in their apartment. The tsunami was rolling in with Jan sitting on its crest. How could she possibly come down to earth and write a meaningful speech? She also knew there was no way she could stand on that stage, looking at the audience, ready to give her speech without causing an earthquake twice the magnitude of the one in 1906!

* * *

Jan sat at her tiny desk fidgeting with her pen as thoughts reeled through her mind so fast they blurred her vision. The stress of writing her speech was driving her crazy. She almost knocked her chair over, as she decided to walk down to Mandy's room.

"Well, hello, sweetness. To what may I contribute this visit from her majesty?"

"Oh Mandy, I'm going wild trying to settle on a few thoughts for my speech."

"What do you have so far?"

"Nothing but a blank page."

"What are some of your ideas?"

"Telling what our training involves, what it's like to be a student nurse. I don't know."

"Jan, calm down. Why don't you tell some true stories about our instructors or us that would make people laugh?"

"Hmm, not a bad idea. Do you have anything funny to tell?"

"How about the time I went to give a patient an intramuscular injection in his buttock, and as I pulled his skin taut with one hand and came down with the needle in the other, it went right through the thin flap of skin holding my thumb on?"

"That's right, and you went ahead and pushed the fluid in and walked away like nothing had happened!"

"How about your highly publicized elevator ride?"

"Okay, Mandy, you have me going. I don't know why you're not giving this talk; our grades were the same."

"Because you're the queen and I'm just your hand maiden. I wouldn't try to walk in your shoes for a trillion dollars; besides your shoe would only fit my big toe!"

"Mandy, you're so funny. Thank you again and again," Jan said as she ran down the hall.

Within a couple of hours, Jan had her talk almost ready. She set it aside and went to lunch with Mandy and the other girls. They discussed the dresses each would wear following graduation. They would be dressed in white dress uniforms for the ceremony. They could change afterwards to their fancy dresses.

Cindy turned to Jan. "Hey, Miss Winston, what are your colors for the wedding?"

"Pale blue and rose, but that reminds me, would anyone like to help me with the decorations for the reception?"

Most of the girls said yes, but a few would be leaving for their hometowns after graduation and wouldn't be able to return. Mandy, Cindy and Kim were to be her bridesmaids, and Jan's sister was her maid of honor.

Jan returned to her room, read her speech and made changes as she went. Since it was Sunday, and Allen was working the full day to give his boss a break, the girls decided to meet in the living room together to study for finals. When they finished, Cindy grabbed Jan and said, "Please come down to my room; I really need to talk to you alone."

"Sure, Cindy. Mandy, I'll be awhile, but we'll go to dinner together, okay?"

"Yeah, no problem."

Cindy and Jan walked down to Cindy's room and made themselves comfortable. "Jan I have something I need to talk about but only if you promise it won't be told to anyone else, ever, ever!"

"Of course, Cindy, you know I don't listen and tell."

"I know, but this is really bad."

"Okay."

"I've been dating a guy for the last six months. As you know, I had stopped dating because I was tired of being used and I was practicing, ah, what did you call it?"

"Celibacy or chastity?"

"Yeah, that's it. When I started dating him, I told him I would not have sex outside of marriage and he said that was fine. I guess I should mention he's been married before and he's seven years older."

"Did he have any children?"

"No, thank goodness. He's really a nice guy, very much like Allen, and we have a lot of fun together. We've gone to the movies, dances and just hung out together. He's mentioned how hard it is on him not having sexual relations since he's been married before. But I've stood my ground."

"Good for you, Cindy."

"No, not so good; let me tell you what happened. We went to a party of one of his buddies who was having a birthday. There was a lot of drinking and, Jan, I like to drink once in awhile. We both had way too much to drink and stayed out after curfew. He told me I could come to his place and sleep it off and he would drive me back early Sunday morning. Jan, It's the first time I had gone to his place, I swear!"

"I believe you, Cindy."

"He told me I could sleep in his bed and he would sleep on the couch. He showed me the bed and started kissing me. He got really carried away and I kept pushing him back, telling him to stop, when he put me on the bed and raped me!"

"Oh no, Cindy!"

"Now, I have to be honest, once he was into things, I let him because by then I wanted it, too."

"But Cindy he forced himself on you, didn't he?"

"Yes, definitely at first."

"Then that's rape!"

"I know, but after he apologized, we slept together in the bed."

"And?"

"He got me back to the dorm early, before anyone was awake, and I climbed in one of the windows downstairs and went to bed. That was the time a month ago when I slept in until noon and everyone thought I was sick. In a lot of ways I was, so I just went along with it."

"I remember. It was the Sunday we brought your dinner to you."

"You're right."

"Cindy, what have you done since then?"

"I kept refusing to see him. Then the other night he met me as I came out to catch the bus after school. He handed me some flowers and asked if he could talk to me over dinner. Jan, he cried when he apologized and he told me he's fallen in love with me and wants to marry me after I graduate."

"And what did you tell him?"

"I said I would have to think about it because of what he did to me. So here I am, seeking some worldly advice from my counselor."

"How do you feel about him?"

"Jan, I'm in love with the guy and I really think it was the alcohol that made him go crazy."

"So, are you telling me you want to say yes to his proposal?"

"I think so, but I'm really scared. Because he did force me to have sex."

"Cindy, no matter how you look at it, what he did was wrong."

"Jan, I have an idea. Why don't we go out to dinner on a double date and don't tell Allen anything about this, but maybe you both can get a better picture of what he's really like; then you can give me your insight, okay?"

"If you really want to, we can do that for you."

"How about next Saturday night?"

"Sure, I'll ask Allen."

CHAPTER FORTY

THE PANIC RETURNS

Monday morning, Jan reported to the emergency room for her last rotation. She was taken on the usual tour and assisted on some minor problems until lunch. Allen picked her up to take her to lunch and class, and she told him, "It was almost boring in ER."

"Really? well isn't it the one place in the hospital where you never know what's going to happen next?"

"I suppose so, but if today is any indication, I think I'll study while I'm there."

"Sounds like a wise move."

The next morning, when she entered the room, Jan felt a pulsation of activity. She was handed a suture kit and told to set up and assist a doctor in unit six. She finished her easy assignment, then entered the hall where she had the feeling she'd been thrown to the center of an ant hill with the queen ant shouting out commands. Patients lay on gurneys, moaning in pain with blood on their sheets. A nurse grabbed Jan's arm, "Follow me."

Jan obediently followed as she saw an ambulance driver rush inside with a badly burned man screaming in pain. The driver turned to the nurse and said, "There's two more just like him coming in!"

The nurse turned to Jan and said, "Find an empty room, transfer him, grab a doc and I'll be right down." The nurse ran to the phone, telling the operator to page all available medical staff to report to ER.

As Jan and the driver located a vacant room, she heard a call on the intercom. "All available medical staff, report to emergency room immediately." It wasn't very long before Miss Kingston and two other instructors showed up with a flock of doctors and nurses.

The nurse grabbed Jan again and told her to team with Dr. Rob Shaw and assist him with his patients. She was grateful to be with Rob as she walked up to him. "I'm your new partner."

"Great, Jan. I don't remember your last name."

"Winston, Miss Winston."

"Why don't you get a handful of suture sets. It looks like we've been assigned to the lacerations and fractures. Meet me down the hall in room two."

"Will do."

She set up for the first laceration, and Dr. Shaw asked the patient, "Can you tell us what happened here?"

The patient answered, "Construction people working on a new building at the manufacturing plant where I'm employed caused some kind of huge explosion. It rocked the main part of the plant like a major earthquake. Debris was flying everywhere, including huge pieces of glass and parts of the building. The heat from the explosion made all of us run for cover, and I wouldn't be a bit surprised if some men were severely burned!"

Jan looked at Rob. Now the burned patients made sense. Miss Kingston approached to ask the patient for some basic information so they could keep track of the injured and answer phone calls from family and friends. She then pinned an identification number to his shirt. She told Jan classes were canceled for the day, and the other students had been told to come to ER as soon as they finished their assignments. Jan thought *Good, no finals today!*

Jan had never heard the term "multitasking" but she learned how to do it real quick that day in ER. It was organized bedlam! She and Doctor Shaw sutured everything from two to twelve inch lacerations of varying depths plus several types of fractures along the way. One patient had a punctured jugular vein that oozed blood all over as soon as the medic took the pressure off. Dr. Shaw worked fast to stabilize it with a couple of hemostats while he and Jan ran the patient up to surgery. Upon their return, things slowed down. They ran into Mandy, and not surprising, Rob pitched in alongside her and other nurses doing cleanup.

An ER nurse walked up to them and said, "Dr. Shaw, you don't have to help with the cleanup. We can do it."

"That's okay. I don't mind helping out."

What a good excuse to stay near Mandy; pretty clever, Rob!

By the end of the day they took a head count: 52 patients were treated for various injuries, 6 sent to surgery, 8 admitted, 4 remained critical and 7 had been killed at the scene. All the student nurses finished the cleanup.

Allen heard the news on the radio and when he called the dorm, he tracked Jan down at the pizza parlor. He greeted Rob and Mandy, and they all took turns filling him in on some of the details. Jan asked him, "How would you feel about going on a double date with Cindy and her boyfriend?"

"Sure, when?"

"This Saturday, okay?"

"That will work."

The girls went back to the dorm completely exhausted with that comfortable feeling that only comes from a job well done.

* * *

Cindy made introductions, "David, I'd like you to meet Allen and Jan."

David was very nice looking, about 6' 1" and a muscular physique. He had a full head of dark wavy hair that gave the impression he had just stepped out of a movie set, depicting a character from the Italian Mafia. Shockingly light blue eyes and a cleft chin enhanced his very good looks.

Dave greeted them with a smile and shook Allen's hand. "Nice to meet you. I understand you two are going to be married in a couple of months?"

"It's a little less than two months, but I'm already shaking in my boots!"

"Allen!" Jan moaned.

"Oh, I'm sorry, didn't know you were standing there."

Cindy laughed, "Oh, Allen."

They were shown to a booth. Jan couldn't help but notice David ordered for Cindy without asking her what she wanted and included a mug of beer with two glasses.

"So Dave, what kind of work do you do?" Allen asked.

"I'm unemployed at the moment. I'm a butcher by trade and going to law school. What do you do, Allen?"

"I'm in college, studying dentistry and I work part time in a gas station. I've always been interested in law, but I don't think my brain is big enough to hold all you need to know."

"I have to admit, it's a major challenge, but being a dentist would require a pretty big brain as well."

David took several gulps of his beer as he turned his attention to Jan. "I hear you're giving a talk at graduation. Are you planning on telling some juicy stories about your classmates?"

"Hey," he gestured to the waitress, "bring me another pitcher midway thru dinner."

Just the mention of her speech brought a tremor of panic. "Maybe just a few wild tales."

Cindy giggled. "I can hardly wait to hear them."

Jan threw the attention back to Dave. "So how did you learn to become a butcher?"

"I lived with my grandmother, and my uncle owned the local butcher shop. I worked for him through high school. It's okay, but I decided a long time ago I didn't want to be a meat cutter all my life."

They made small talk during dinner, and David managed to drink a tremendous amount of beer to Cindy's one glass. Jan could see a difference in his behavior as the evening progressed.

Allen made a suggestion, "There's a dance hall not too far from here. Would you like to join us in some dancing?"

Cindy said, "Oh Dave, you can't believe what great dancers these two are; we should go just so we can watch."

David answered, "Sounds like fun, but Cindy, you already know, I'm not a bad dancer myself."

"Great, let's go."

They showed up at the dance as the music was playing, and Allen lost no time getting Jan on the dance floor. Jan noticed Cindy and David were sitting at their table absorbed in a deep conversation. She thought. *Why isn't he proving what a great dancer he is, or is he trying to convince her to marry him? Heaven forbid!*

Allen moved her onto the dance floor for a slow dance, and Jan forgot about them as Allen whispered in her ear, "My Pumpkin is deep in thought. Are you thinking about our first dance as Mr. and Mrs. Morris?"

"Oh my goodness, we do have to decide what we'll have them play for our dance together."

"We both love Johnny Mathis. How about something he sings?"

"That's perfect, one of our favorites is "Chances Are.""

"For now, shall we settle for it unless we change our minds?"

After the dance, they walked back to the table. Cindy was smiling from ear to ear.

"Guess what, Dave asked me to marry him. And I said yes."

Allen asked, "When do you intend to get married?"

"As soon as possible after I graduate and have a job."

Jan sat very quietly. *So much for getting our opinion about David. That's Cindy, impulsively jumping in. Well, maybe I can talk some sense into her later.*

"Jan, are you excited for me?"

"More like dumbfounded, Cindy."

"I know, me too."

Dave stood up, "I think we'll be on our way now. Nice meeting you." He pulled her to the door.

After they left, Allen wanted to dance, and Jan said, "Can we talk for a minute?"

"Sure, Pumpkin."

"How did you feel about David?"

"Well, other than drinking a bit too much, he seemed like a nice enough guy. Why?"

"I don't feel good about him. Yes, he's nice, but there's just something about him, I don't know."

"And I think you worry too much about your friends. She's old enough to make her own decisions, besides, if she makes the wrong one, you'll be there to help her pick up the pieces, right?"

"Yes, I guess you have a point there."

"Now can we dance?"

"Beat you to the dance floor."

* * *

Alone in her room, Jan was in the middle of reading her talk aloud when Mandy walked in asking, "Jan, would you like to try it out on me? I'll be happy to give you a second opinion."

"Okay, close the door so others won't hear. I want them to be surprised."

As she read out loud, Jan made a few changes along the way. Mandy also timed her so she would know if it fit in the time allotted. When she finished, Mandy said, "Jan it's great. You really did a super job. Are you going to be all right when you get up in front of everyone?"

"Oh Mandy, my panic just surfaced as you asked me that. I don't know how I'll be."

"I believe we'll be sitting in the front row, so if you want, just talk directly to me. I'll be there for you. You know I will, don't you?"

"Yes, of course I do. In the next few weeks, I'm going to try to memorize it so I don't have to read it. I'll feel less panic by telling it off the top of my head."

"You have a typewriter on your head?"

"Oh Mandy, let's go to lunch and we can study for this week's finals."

When Mandy and Jan entered the hall, Cindy grabbed Jan saying, "We need to talk."

"Can't it wait until after lunch? I'm starved. Why don't you join us for lunch and then we'll talk."

"Oh, okay. Let's go."

When they returned, Jan went with Cindy to her room. Cindy asked, "Tell me what Allen said about David."

"Well, other than drinking too much, he seems like a nice enough guy. I definitely have some reservations about him, Cindy."

Cindy sounded a bit defensive. "Like what?"

"I get the impression he will want to keep you under his thumb, telling you what you can and can't do. And he drinks a lot."

"Oh Jan, he only drinks like that on the weekends when we go out. He doesn't drink at all during the week."

"Okay, why did he order for you at the restaurant without asking you what you wanted?"

"He always does that. I think it's so neat!"

"Well, if you don't mind, that's fine. I have to admit, it would really bother me."

"Oh. Well, thanks for talking to me. Guess we should study."

CHAPTER FORTY ONE

THE GRADUATION GIFT

Graduation was within a few days. Janet had just finished her last day in ER. Thank goodness they never had a repeat of her second day. She learned later, two of the burn victims had died, and the other one was slowly healing. She enjoyed the fast pace of ER, but when it dragged, it was boring. The hardest ones to deal with were the little children. Many toddlers brought in with raspy breathing, running a temp and would end up in surgery with a peanut or a jelly bean in their lungs. One she would never forget had a sharp pencil stuck in his chest. Luckily the mother didn't try to pull it out, he would have bled to death because it had pierced his aorta! An eight year old ran into a closed patio door, breaking the glass, and had some severe lacerations. Jan returned to the dorm with another bloody apron after tending that child.

In their nursing classes they had been given pointers for state boards along with obsolete tests to study by. The class members went shopping for white dress uniforms to wear at graduation. Jan had but one objective during this time and that was to have her speech behind her. She practiced in front of her mirror countless times both with and then without her papers, but each time the Mexican jumping beans would disturb her digestion. Allen and Mandy gave her words of encouragement; she only wished she felt more courageous herself.

* * *

Jan pulled the covers around her like a baby seal tucked inside her mother's flippers. It was impossible to sleep knowing what was coming in the morning. *Maybe I can pretend I'm sick. How about a migraine? I've never had one before, so I wouldn't know how to act. Let me think of something else. I know; I was throwing up all night. It's no use. I can't lie. Besides, I don't want to miss my graduation. I've worked three years for this! You can do this Jan. You made it through the skit, and you gave a talk at the grammar school about patriotism to earn your grade in public speaking. You just have to get a hold of yourself. Maybe I should say a prayer. Will He hear me? I'll try "Please, Lord, help me be calm for my speech and remember what I've prepared. I do believe in you, but I don't know if you will listen to me. I guess that's all."*

Jan experienced a feeling of warmth, as a sense of calm swept over her. She turned on her side, said "Thank you" and went fast asleep. In the morning, she woke up feeling great. She took her shower and Mandy came down to do her hair. Jan told her what had happened the night before.

Mandy said, "Really? Maybe I should try praying or something. I'm nervous about walking across the stage to receive my diploma. I keep visualizing myself tripping over my own over-sized feet and taking a header!"

"Mandy, you're going to be just fine. Don't forget, you and Rob are invited to Aunt Barbara's for a celebration after the ceremony."

"Do we have to wear our uniforms?"

"Not if you stay for pictures with me after. Then we can rush back to the dorm and change."

"Oh, good."

"You did invite Rob, right?"

"Well of course. I wouldn't come without him!"

Jan laughed at Mandy. "And I'm glad to hear that. Cindy and David plus Kim with her boyfriend are going to come."

Mandy said, "Sounds like this will be quite a party. Did I tell you I have an interview on Monday?"

"For the third time! Now just make sure they will give you the day of the wedding off. My interview's Tuesday morning."

"See, you do it too. You told me yesterday."

"Okay, Mandy. We're even. Would you mind if I run through my speech once again while my hair is drying?"

"Okay, I mind. Go ahead, and then I'll do your nails and makeup."

Jan ran through it real fast, looking at her notes only twice.

"You did that in record time. Slow down a little and you'll do just fine. Remember, I believe in you."

"I know you do, and I love you so much for being my best friend."

"I love me too. Oh no, I love *you* too."

* * *

Jan was quiet as Allen drove her to the campus. "I didn't know you could ever be speechless, Pumpkin. Are you okay?"

"I will be when I finish my talk. Did you know I have to sit on the stage with all the dignitaries?"

"Of course. That's because you're 'sooo' special."

"Only to you, Allen."

"You're so funny."

"Funny how?"

"You are special to everyone, not just to your parents and not just to me. You're an extraordinary woman. Do you think I would be marrying you if you weren't?"

"Thank you, Allen, but I think you're wearing rose-colored glasses."

He pulled up to the auditorium and Jan jumped out so she could find her place with the graduating nurses. They would be the first to enter; then the college grads would follow them.

As they marched in to the music of 'Pomp and Circumstance,' Jan's heart started to pound, and for a moment she felt her emotions getting the best of her. To gain control of herself, she focused on moving her feet to the rhythm of the music. She looked ahead at the stage and couldn't believe she had to sit with all of those important people. She still felt remarkably peaceful with just a few mild tremors. Absent was the major "Don Knott's geological phenomenon!" She took her seat and looked out on the audience. *Where did all those people come from; it's filled to capacity and people are lining up against the walls. This is incredible; they should have held this in the stadium.*

The college grads were entering now. She kept looking for Allen. Finally, she saw him. It seemed like such a long time before he appeared. When he entered, he looked right at her, never taking his eyes off her until he sat down. She was filled with confidence as she anticipated her speech.

The college president was the master of ceremonies and when he called Janet's name, a slight tremor surged through her body. She took her place at the podium and recognized the dignitaries. Jan then paused while she looked upon the audience. "I would like to introduce an important, honored guest and request she join me. Miss Kingston, please?" Jan made a gesture for her to come to the podium.

As Jan looked up at Miss Kingston, she said, "Ladies and gentlemen, I want you to know that we have just completed three years under the watchful eye of this elegant lady standing beside me. Our first year, she taught us the true meaning of terror when she was in our presence. Well look at her-she's at least two feet taller than I! Miss Kingston actually chuckled. The second year we began to realize there might be a beating heart behind this impenetrable wall surrounding her. And by the third year we grew to appreciate the great human being she truly is and how much we have been able to learn under her direction. On behalf of your 1960 graduating class, we would like you to accept this plaque in your honor."

The audience gave her a standing ovation. As Jan looked out at everyone, she spotted Mrs. Stewart standing in the back wiping tears from her face. She was sincerely happy to see Miss Kingston's sister there.

Miss Kingston was too emotional to say anything but "thank you" and sat back down. Jan continued, "We've had many experiences through these years, some emotionally draining, some I don't dare repeat in mixed company, and others hysterically funny. One of the students sitting in front of me stuck the needle through part of her hand when giving an injection. Another slipped while carrying a full bedpan and ended up going back to the nurse's dorm to take a shower and change her uniform. We could smell her coming and going for days after. Many of us, while learning to shake a glass thermometer down, had it flip out of our hands, crash to the floor where it emptied its contents. Have you ever tried to pick mercury up from the floor? I made front page news when I almost died while stuck in the hospital elevator, but my notoriety didn't stop there; while in the psych ward, one of the patients decided I needed an attitude adjustment and fractured my nose." Reaching up to touch her nose, Jan added, "I think I just found my new attitude."

Jan didn't think once of her panic. Her timing was perfect. She waited for laughter to die down before speaking again. Looking at her notes only briefly, she continued, "We have spent quality time in every aspect of nursing. Through the skillful eyes of our dedicated instructors, we've been molded into the kind of nurses anyone would want at their bedside. The kind of nurse a surgeon would prefer to be his assistant and the nurse capable of delivering a baby in bed when mom decides she can't wait for the doctor! We've been taught the art of compassion, of anticipating needs before they're spoken, of improvising when supplies are missing and of giving love when love is all that's left to give.

These seventeen nurses sitting in front of me are the cream of the crop. We started with 54 students. Yes, we lost two thirds of the original nurses enrolled, but these remaining will make a difference in the lives of their patients. They will be applauded by their employers and they'll be loved by their fellow nurses. I have had the privilege of working beside them. I have watched every one (including myself) grow, mature and blossom into the nurses they are today, and I stand before you with my heart full of humility to be one of them.

Thank you Miss Kingston, Mrs. Jacob, Miss Page, Mrs. Novak and a special thanks to Dr. Lowry. Now we face the biggest challenge of all: passing state boards.

As Jan sat down in the midst of thundering applause her nerves took over and she vibrated like a chain saw cutting through a green log. It lasted about 10 minutes, but as she looked out at the special people in the audience, they each in turn gave her a warming smile. She now knew how to get over her panic attacks and she was close to tears with relief.

Miss Kingston stood with the college president to hand out their diplomas; when Jan's name was called, she received a standing ovation, nearly flooring her. She was amazed at the compliments when the ceremony ended. Her dad hugged her with tears in his eyes. "My little girl, I'm so proud of you." Her mom and sister gave her hugs and compliments.

Finally Allen reached her through the crowd and surrounded her in his arms and gave her a kiss. "I told you you're an awesome lady and you just proved it today. And I'm not wearing rose-colored glasses!"

"Oh, Allen, you always make me feel so good."

His parents interrupted. "Can we break this up and congratulate our daughter to be?"

They both hugged her, and then Frank said, "I'm not sure my son will be capable of living with such a celebrity!"

Allen interrupted, "Oh, I think I can handle it."

She felt an arm around her shoulder, turned, and there stood Carol. "You are something else Miss Jan!"

As Carol hugged her, Jan said, "I'm so happy you came. I tried to call you to invite you to the party afterward, but you never answered."

"I'd love to come and I received your invitation to the wedding. I wouldn't miss it for a new Buick!"

Jan pulled her towards Barb. "Would you give my friend Carol directions so she can join us this afternoon?"

"Sure."

Just then she saw Mrs. Stewart standing a few feet in front of her, looking like she was petrified to come any closer. Jan said, "Mrs. Stewart, I'm happy to see you."

She slowly came forward and shook Jan's hand. "Congratulations, and thank you for honoring my sister." As soon as she had spoken to Jan, she turned and rushed into the crowd.

Jan hollered after her, "Well, thank you!" as her dad called for her to take pictures.

Barb outdid herself with a huge cake displaying a nurses' cap and mortar board and big letters reading, "CONGRATULATIONS TO THE GRADUATES."

At one point Frank worked his way over to Jan and gave her a hug. Stepping back with his hands on both of her shoulders, he said, "Jan, I couldn't be happier to have you for the daughter we were unable to have. If I dropped dead tomorrow, I would die a happy man, knowing you'll be taking good care of my wonderful son!"

With all these compliments, Jan feared she may never be able to meet everyone's high expectations. It scared her half to death. She knew she'd been set on top of that pedestal again; and as she teetered there, it made her wonder when it would be kicked out from under her.

During the party, Jan's dad asked for everyone's attention. "From what I've been told, it's customary to give the graduate a gift. And in this case, we have a gift to be shared by both our graduates-our daughter and our son to be."

Jan's mother walked up and handed them both a very small box wrapped in school colors. Allen said, "Jan, you go first."

Her dad said, "No, I think it's best for you to open the boxes at the same time."

Their curiosity had peeked to the top of Mt. Everest by then. They unwrapped the boxes, taking the lids off at the same time. They both held up a pair of car keys. Jan screamed and Allen hollered, "Whoa!"

Jan was first out the door with Allen right behind her. She squealed as they saw a brand- new light blue Ford parked in the driveway. Jan opened the door with her key and slid behind the driver's seat, turning the key in the ignition. Allen jumped into the passenger seat. She rolled the window down, took hold of the gear shift and put the car in reverse. She waved goodbye to her folks. She took off down the quiet neighborhood street. "OH MY HEAVENS TO BETSY. HIP! HIP! HURRAY! WHEE! WE'VE GOT A NEW COVERED WAGON! I'M READY TO DRAG RACE!"

"Have you flipped your lid? If I didn't know better, I'd think you're drunk. And when are you going to let your best friend get behind the wheel?" asked Allen.

Jan made a U turn as she said, "I'll go right back and get Mandy." At the same time, she applied the brakes, throwing them both forward in their seats.

She jumped out, letting Allen slide under the steering wheel while Jan sat in the passenger seat.

Allen looked at her like she'd gone completely and totally insane then burst out laughing as he drove away. "You are a nut case, you know that? I'm going to marry a crazy woman! And I thought I was your best friend."

"Well, maybe."

Allen pulled into the driveway, and ran into the house. They jumped up and down saying, "Thank you, thank you, thank you!"

Jan hugged her dad saying, "This solves our problem of going in two directions at once with Allen in college and me working. You have no idea what a wonderful gift this is."

Her dad answered, "Jan, ever since you gave back the small car I gave you when you started this adventure, I sold it and saved the money with this graduation gift in mind. You and Allen are certainly worth helping out, and we kind of figured you would have a bit of a problem with transportation once you were married."

Allen spoke up, "We had talked about buying an old clunker to keep us going, or one of us taking public transportation, but this is much better and we do appreciate it. My only hope is Jan will let me drive it once in awhile."

CHAPTER FORTY TWO
THE DREADED PHONE CALL

The students were given the following week to vacate the nurse's dormitory. Aunt Barb asked Jan if she would like to stay with her until the wedding. She gladly accepted, so she packed some of her stuff to go to the apartment and just enough of her clothes and personal items to go to Aunt Barb's.

Allen packed up their new car and they went together to the apartment to unload. While he was bringing things in, Jan went through making a list of things they needed to start their life together. The apartment was one of four in an older Victorian home that had been remodeled. They all used the same ornate front door, then each had their own entrance-two upstairs and two down. Jan and Allen had a small living room, dining room with a fold up bed behind a wide closet door, one bathroom, a bedroom and kitchen. They even had a tiny back porch. They were both excited about their little place and could hardly wait to occupy it together. The place was furnished, so all they needed to buy was a combination radio and phonograph player so they could dance.

They hesitated before leaving. Allen took Jan in his arms, kissed her passionately and said, "It won't be long before we can . . ."

"Don't say it Allen. We'll be tempted!"

"You silly, I was going to say, 'We can have water fights in our own apartment.'"

"Are you sure you were going to say that?"

"I'll never tell. But from now until we're married, we need to bring a chaperone with us."

They laughed and went out the door. On the way back to the dorm, Jan asked, "Did I tell you Mandy was offered a job this morning starting on Wednesday as a surgical nurse?"

"That's wonderful. Your interview's tomorrow, isn't it?"

"It sure is! And Mandy's allowed to live in one of the little places behind the Children's Home.

Oh, and Dave found a job in a local market, so they'll be getting married soon. Cindy asked if we would stand up with them at the local Justice of the Peace; I took the liberty to say yes."

"Oh, so now you're going to speak for me?"

"You bet I am."

"Not until you're Mrs. Morris, Miss Winston."

"Ha, just try and stop me."

Allen pulled over, reaching across the gear shift, and kissed her. "Now you should stay quiet for awhile."

"I bet I won't. Take me back to the dorm. I have a few more things to pick up, and then I'll move in with Aunt Barb. She told me we can go shopping together to pick up things for the reception and stuff for the apartment. Then she'll help me decorate the apartment. I just adore your aunt!"

"Yeah, she's pretty special." He pulled in front of the dorm. Here we are, do you need help?"

"Not really. You need to get to the gas station, right?"

"Yep."

Just then, Cindy was running towards the car all excited. "I have great news! I have a job in labor and delivery starting next Monday and Dave wants to get married tomorrow. Can you make it?"

Jan answered, "As long as it's in the early afternoon; my interview's in the morning."

Cindy jumped up and down. "I'm going to call Dave right now!"

Allen looked at Cindy seriously. "Cindy before you do, may I have a word with you?"

Cindy asked, "You aren't going to try talking me out of this, are you?"

"I just want to ask you a couple of questions, that's all."

She leaned on the open window, and Allen said, "Cindy, have you ever met David's parents?"

"No, they've been divorced, and he lost track of his dad since he's been in and out of prison. His mom left him at his grandmother's when he was 10. He doesn't know where she is, and his grandma died a couple of years ago."

"Have you visited your parents with him?"

"No, I pretty much divorced them when I left for college."

"Do you know anything about his previous marriage?"

"Just that she was a nut case and he caught her in bed with another man. Allen, why are you asking me all these questions? I feel like I'm on the hot seat or something."

"I'm sorry, Cindy; I didn't mean to make you feel that way."

"That's okay, but now I really need to go upstairs and pack."

"Okay." Allen kissed Jan, stepped over to his VW and went off to work. Jan loaded the new car and drove to Aunt Barb's.

* * *

Janet Winston walked into Mrs. Caspar's office, they shook hands and Jan took a seat opposite the director's desk.

"Miss Winston, I want you to know how much I enjoyed your speech at graduation. You are a gifted speaker, and what you did for Miss Kingston was priceless."

"Thank you."

"Miss Winston, I have been holding back from filling an available position until I talked to you."

"Really. What is it?"

"It's the position of a 'float nurse'. The reason I want to offer this to you is because you seem to adjust well to change. Not everyone can do that. Do you know what a 'float' does?"

"I believe they go wherever there's a need, but I'm not sure how it works."

"This is the way it's done. The nursing staff always lets my office know when a nurse calls in sick or time off is scheduled. So the float reports to this office and one of my assistants tells her where she's assigned. It can be anywhere in the hospital: the specialized services in the wings or the children's home. The time spent in one place can be anywhere from one day to a month or so. Do you have any questions?"

"Will I be considered for a permanent opening, if one comes up?"

"Absolutely. Do you have a preference?"

"Yes I do. I'd love to spend more time in Pediatrics, especially the Burn Unit."

"I will certainly keep that in mind. Now, Miss Winston, when can you start?"

"I'm sure you already know about my wedding, which is just around the corner. Our honeymoon will be the following week."

Mrs. Caspar looked at her surprised. "You're getting married? I had no idea. Does Miss Kingston know?"

"Well, yes, she received an invitation, and I sent you one also. They were mailed over a month ago."

Mrs. Caspar got out of her chair and went to her secretary. "Faye, would you check through the mail and see if I have anything from Miss Winston? And if not, go down to the mail room to see if it's been misplaced."

Jan jumped up and told the secretary, "It's in a pale blue envelope."

Faye said, "I'll get right on it."

They went back in her office and Mrs. Caspar spoke first. "Well, this changes things a bit. I'm sure you don't want to work at all before the wedding."

"It would make it really hard. There's so much to do, unless you really need me."

"It's not a problem. We'll make up a name tag for you with your married name. What will it be?"

"Morris."

"Janet Morris? Okay. What I've done with the other students is give them a temporary name tag with GN (graduate nurse) at the end of their name. You'll all be issued a regular one once you've received your RN license. So your starting date will be the Monday after your honeymoon. Will that work for you?"

Faye came running in waving the invitation. "It had fallen behind the wire rack in the mail room, and mail received since then covered it."

Mrs. Caspar neatly took her letter opener and pulled out the invitation. "Oh, this is lovely. I'm excited for you. And I'm so glad it's local; I'll be able to make it. Is it alright to bring my husband?"

"Oh, of course it is."

"Thank you, Miss Winston, and make sure you fill out all the paperwork with my secretary on your way out. I'll see on your wedding day."

"Thank you so much, Mrs. Caspar."

Jan ran out to Aunt Barb who was taking in a lovely late spring day sunning herself on the lawn in front of her car. She jumped up when she saw Jan. "Did you get the job?"

"No, she told me I wasn't good enough to work here."

"Oh, you are full of it, young lady! Where will you be assigned?"

"I'm going to be a float for now. I'll explain while we drive home."

"All right. Can hardly wait to help you pick out your going-away outfit and some curtains for your kitchen. The ones they have in your apartment look a hundred years old. Do you think we'll have enough time when you get back from the ceremony?"

"I'm pretty sure. They're being married by a justice of the peace, so it shouldn't take too long. Then we'll probably take them out for a quick celebration."

* * *

Allen and Jan drove quietly to the home of the justice of the peace. The couple was waiting for them in front. Cindy ran to their car and said, "We're so excited, we can hardly stand it."

"Wonderful, Cindy, shall we go in?" Allen said.

Jan tried very hard to put on a happy face for Cindy's benefit as they entered and were introduced to the officiator. The gentleman gave a very nice talk about the marriage commitment, then he asked them the regular questions and pronounced them 'Man and Wife,' Dave kissed Cindy long and hard until he heard someone clear his throat, then they stopped. Congratulations were in order, then Allen invited them out to celebrate and they readily accepted.

Allen asked, "Do you have a favorite restaurant?"

Cindy said, "I'm craving pizza."

"Do you know where the Zombie Zulu Hut is?"

David answered, "I've driven by there but never gone in. Is it good?"

"Jan and I love their pizza."

"Okay, we'll meet you there."

The foursome ordered Dave and Cindy's favorite then the newly married couple guzzled beer like they were terrified it was about to be abolished from the country. The newlyweds left as soon as they ate, refusing Allen's offer to drive them home.

Allen leaned forward as he held a piece of pizza mid air. "As I said before and I'm saying it again, I have to admit I kind of like Dave."

"I do too, Allen. I can't explain why I have such an uneasy feeling about them."

"Okay, enough said. Now I need to get you back to your guardian. She said you're going shopping, right?"

* * *

Jan and Barb had such fun together. The time flew by and they came back with everything she needed. She chose a dress with a floral print of pale yellow and orange flowers on an off-white background which came with a linen cloak and a wide brimmed hat, all matching the colors in the dress. "Jan, you look absolutely stunning in your outfit --- perfect to wear to a fancy hotel downtown," said Barb.

Jan blushed at the mention of the hotel. She took in a deep breath and broached the subject with Aunt Barb. "I'm absolutely terrified of my wedding night, Aunt Barb."

"Well, I can certainly relate to how you're feeling, Jan. I was so frightened I stayed in the bathroom for two hours trying to work up the nerve to go into the bedroom. My husband kept coming to the door asking me if I was alright. Poor guy, he was worried sick."

"What was it like when you came out?"

"I told him how frightened I was. Then he told me he was scared also. We started to laugh together, then we kissed. Before we knew it, nature took its course. Just relax, Jan; it's really a beautiful experience. And it brings the two of you close in a way that binds your marital commitment."

"Thanks, Aunt Barb, I needed to hear that."

The phone rang. Jan ran out to the car to bring in the rest of the bags and Barb went to answer it. Jan walked back into the house, took one look at Aunt Barb and knew something terrible had just happened! She felt a chill as she threw her packages down. "What's wrong, what is it?"

CHAPTER FORTY THREE
HOW CAN THIS BE HAPPENING NOW?

With a shaky voice Barb spoke. "Carmela just called. Oh I can't believe it!" She stood there, wringing her hands with a handkerchief. "Frank, he," Barb began to sob out of control.

Janet put her arm around her. "It's okay. Come sit down; try to catch your breath and tell me what she said."

She blew her nose and in an unsteady voice answered, "Frank has had a severe heart attack and Carm said we better get Allen and come up immediately. Will you call Allen please?"

"Barb, get some things together, and we can drive over to the apartment. Allen was going to repair a few things there, and I think it's best to tell him in person. We can leave from there."

When they walked into the apartment, Allen was carrying some tools into the dining room. He took one look at them and set the tools on the table, saying, "What in the world is wrong?"

Jan quietly took his hand and said, "Your dad." Allen gasped. "Your dad has had a heart attack, and we need to drive up immediately!"

The three of them walked out of the apartment in a stupor. How could something happen now at the happiest time of their lives? They needed Frank to be at their wedding. He was Allen's best man, and they wanted him to be around as a grandfather to their children.

They drove pretty much in silence, each absorbed in his or her own thoughts. Allen pulled into the parking lot of the hospital and opened the car doors for them. They walked into the hospital, and the receptionist said, "He's in room 103, Allen, your mom's expecting you."

Allen's mom rushed to him, bursting out in tears. "Doctor says he's had a massive heart attack and there's nothing more they can do!"

Jan gravitated to Frank's bedside, doing a silent evaluation (wishing she had brought her stethoscope with her). He was unresponsive and displayed the classic signs of impending death. She knew it was a matter of hours, if not sooner. *Why Lord, why now when he had turned his life around and we need him to be a part of our family. This just isn't right!*

Jan turned back to Allen and his mom, hugging her then Allen. He looked down at her and asked, "What do you think? Is he going to make it?"

"Oh, Allen, it really doesn't look good. I think you should go over and talk to him. Tell him how much you love him or what's in your heart to say. He will hear every word. We know the last sense to go is hearing."

Mom heard what Jan said. "I'm so glad to hear that; I've been pouring my heart out to him ever since he was brought to his room."

Allen walked over to his bedside, took his dad's hand in his and quietly talked to him.

After a few minutes the doctor walked in, listened to Frank's heart then turned to the family. "I'm sorry, I don't think it will be more than a few hours. His heart is badly damaged and he's weakening rapidly. I wish there was something I could do, but it's out of my hands now."

Allen looked like a puppy shrinking away from a severe beating. The pain was far too much to absorb and he stood there shaking his head, looking down at the floor. They had had so little time together since his recovery. They were looking forward to being together after the honeymoon, before Allen's university classes began.

Jan wrapped her arms around Allen and they stood together feeling the energy of profound grief shared between them. His mother had moved over to Frank's beside. Suddenly she spoke. "Allen and Jan come over here quick. I think he's leaving us!"

They came to the bedside. He looked so peaceful. Jan felt for a pulse. There was none. Aunt Barb who had watched stoically until now, put a hand to each side of her face and began sobbing as she backed away from his bed. Allen went to her side and held her in his arms. Jan moved to his mom and put her arms around her as they silently wept together. It was so sudden, the reality seemed more than any one of them could endure.

They heard someone clear his throat, and Peter Savio, the sheriff, was standing in the doorway. "I'm sorry if I'm interrupting. I can come back; I just heard the news and had to come."

Allen went over, extending his hand as he said, "Pete, he just now died."

Pete grabbed Allen in a bear hug. "I'm so sorry. How can this be happening? I just talked to him two days ago, telling him the latest on the fugitives. As we talked he looked so healthy and was excitedly telling me about the pending wedding. I just can't believe it!"

Allen took Peter aside and asked, "Pete, what did you tell my dad about the brothers?"

"They've been spotted a couple of times buying supplies in a little town on the Nevada/ California state line. We think they're hiding out in the mountains above your family cabin. We plan a combined search of several law enforcement agencies to try to flush them out."

"Pete, we're spending our honeymoon at the cabin. Is it safe?"

"I'm sure it is. They're staying real secluded. We suspect they're up around Peep Sight Rock. From up there they can see all sides below if anyone approaches. We're planning our approach in the next week or so, at first dawn, hoping they'll be asleep."

The nurses came in telling them the doctor was on his way. Pete gave Carmela a hug and said, "Please call me if I can do anything. I would like to offer some of my men as pall bearers unless you have someone else in mind. And if you'd like, we will give him a law enforcement funeral with all the honors; he really deserves it."

"Pete, I'm sure Frank would want that. I'll let you know when the mortuary can schedule it."

Within minutes of the sheriff leaving the doctor walked in, checked him with his stethoscope. Turning to Carmela he said, "It's always hardest on the family when they go so fast, but that's most likely what Frank ordered."

Carmela whimpered, "He has told me many times since his suffering in the mine shaft, he would rather drop dead than linger. Once was enough for him. I know the Lord blessed him by granting him his wish."

The doctor turned to Allen. "Is this the student nurse you told us about?"

"Yes, my bride this next Saturday."

"Well, Frank sure picked a heck of a time to pull his stunt; but he would want you to go through with your plans and enjoy your life together. Why don't you kids go over to the mortuary to help your mom. We'll get him ready to be picked up."

The four of them walked out, their steps on automatic as Allen turned to Jan and said, "I'll drive Mom over; you and Barb can follow me."

Jan was so worried about Allen. He looked like a rag doll without his stuffing-powerless to fight the feeling of his loss. Would he be able to come out of it in time for the wedding? Jan wasn't so sure.

* * *

Barb and Jan drove home together, leaving Allen to help his mom. Janet focused on doing as much as possible before this unexpected wedge was placed in her time frame. The final fitting of her wedding dress was moved up to Wednesday instead of Thursday now that the funeral was able to be scheduled on that day. As the dress was zippered in the back, the attendant said she must have lost a couple of pounds, so she would need to take it in a bit. Jan gingerly removed the gown to avoid the pins, and they assured her it could be picked up Saturday morning.

Jan's mom arrived to help out and the three of them shopped together to buy clothes appropriate for the funeral. Jan didn't have a black dress in her closet. The excitement of the wedding was suddenly dampened, like putting a cover on a boiling pot and moving it off the burner. The shock and sadness of dealing with the reality of the pending funeral was palpable.

When morning came it was difficult to prepare for what they knew lay ahead for the day. Leaving before dawn, Jan drove her car with Barb. Jan's parents followed in their automobile. It was so quiet, Jan needed to think of happier thoughts as she asked Aunt Barbara, "Would you like to hear about our future plans after the wedding?"

"I'd love that, dear."

"While Allen finishes his education, I'll continue to work as our primary means of support. Allen will then have to do his internship. Once he establishes his own practice, I'll continue to work until I get pregnant, then I'll be a housewife until they're in school."

"Sounds like you have everything well planned. Just a word to the wise. Something always seems to happen when you least expect it, forcing you to take a detour around those well laid-out plans."

"I suppose so. We'll just have to build a temporary bridge when the river washes our designs away."

They went directly to Carmela's home where she was busy getting serving dishes prepared for the gathering afterward. She had a local chef catering the food for the expected crowd, since everyone in town knew Frank. Jan and Barb pitched in immediately.

Carmela spoke to Barbara regarding her plans following the funeral. "Barb, if you don't mind, after the funeral, I'd like you to drive me down in my car. That way, I can help these youngsters with their preparations."

Barb answered, "Carm, I would love to have you stay for as long as you like after the wedding; I can use the company and I'm sure you can, too. Then I'd be happy to come up and help you with things up here."

Allen had an idea. "We can come to Aunt Barb's when we return from our honeymoon and open our wedding gifts with you."

"That's sounds great. Allen and Jan, would you like to invite some of your friends over also?" Barb asked.

"Yes, I especially want Mandy over, and maybe Cindy and Kim. Oh and Carol, too." Jan said.

"Allen, what time is it?" his mother asked.

Allen glanced at his watch. "It's time to get dressed. The mortuary limousine will be here in less than 30 minutes Mom."

Jan glanced at Barb. "We get to ride in a limo?"

"Yes, honey. It's provided for the immediate family at most funerals."

"Well, I guess that's why I didn't know. I've never been to a family funeral before."

Barb patted her hand. "I'm sorry you had to do it a few days before your wedding, dear."

They sat quietly in the limousine as they rode into town. Allen held her hand so tight it hurt but she wasn't about to let go. She knew he was hanging on for dear life, afraid he would break down.

Jan was shocked to see police officers lining the street as they drove in. It was so moving, she felt the tears rise and spill down her cheeks.

The sheriff and another officer, both in dress uniform, opened the doors for them. They were ushered in through a private entrance to a room reserved for family and invited guests. Organ music was playing, and from their viewpoint they could see the casket. A minister started the ceremony, then, to her surprise, Allen was asked to say a few words.

Before stepping to the podium, Allen stopped and glanced at his dad. Janet held her breath, so afraid he'd break down. When he spoke, his voice was strong and calm. He talked about his dad's life, his accomplishments and his near-death experience at the bottom of a mine shaft. He purposely left out his years of darkness. He told them what a great husband and father he'd been and the kinds of lessons he taught him. He closed by saying his mother had made a special request for him to sing one of his father's favorite hymns. The organ started playing; he adjusted the microphone and sang, "God Be With You 'til We Meet Again." He had a lovely tenor voice, and Jan was shocked, once again, to learn something new about him just a few days before marriage. She had heard him sing in church but had no idea his voice was so beautiful.

He returned, taking his seat quietly between Jan and his mother. Jan didn't dare say anything, even though she was exploding inside with the knowledge that he was such a great big surprise package. The rest of the funeral went well. Jan broke down as she stood before Frank in his casket. Reality hit her and Allen held her in his arms as they sobbed together.

When they approached the cemetery, the police officers stood at attention on both sides of the road leading to his grave site. The sheriff officiated and his talk about Frank was remarkably uplifting. They said their goodbyes, then many followed them to the ranch.

Jan and Barb busied themselves in the kitchen cleaning dishes and refilling them with the catered food, so Mom and Allen were free to greet people. Even though the house was very large, there was standing room only as people continued to arrive. As Jan was arranging the table, she watched Allen as he walked through the crowd. The perfect host uplifted others with hugs and warm greetings as he went. She realized he was working his way over to her, and when he arrived at the table, he put his arms around her, kissed her lightly and said, "How's my Pumpkin doing?"

"I'm doing fine. How about you?"

"I'm good. I've had the distinct impression he's been here with us. Is that too weird?"

"No. Barb and I were talking about it in the kitchen, and we've been feeling the same thing."

"Wow. I'll bet Mom has, too."

"I'm sure she has."

An elderly couple walked up behind them. "Allen, is this your beautiful bride?"

"Yes, I'd like you to meet Janet Winston."

"Isn't the wedding this weekend?"

"Yes, it is"

"Well, shame on Frank for doing this to you just before getting married!"

Allen smiled. "Better now than during our honeymoon."

The lady giggled. "Oh, you're so right."

They walked away, and Allen whispered, "I couldn't remember their names to introduce you."

"It's okay; I probably wouldn't remember anyway. Now I'd better help Aunt Barb in the kitchen."

On the drive home Jan said, "What other surprises do you have in store for me, Mr. Morris?"

"I'll never tell."

"Do you realize what a total shock it was to me when you sang a solo?"

"Do you know what a total shock you were to me when you gave your talk?"

"Oh, are you saying we're even?"

"I guess you'll find out in a couple of days. Speaking of that, I would like our dance song to be 'The Twelfth of Never' by Johnny Mathis instead of 'Chances Are'. What do you think?"

"I think that's perfect. It's a slow waltz you know?"

"Why do you think I made that suggestion?"

He pulled up in front of the apartment. "Do you want to come in?"

"Yes, you can help me hang the kitchen curtains, okay?"

"Okay, and you can make me a list of things I can do to help."

"Don't you have to work?"

"No, my boss got his son to help out because of what happened, and I don't have to go back to work until the same day you do."

"I'm so happy; you can help with a whole lot of stuff."

When they were inside, Allen turned her around, kissing her tenderly and as he held her in his embrace he said, "Thank you for standing by me today and helping my mom and Aunt Barb."

"It was my pleasure. Now let's get to work."

While Jan was hanging the curtains, Allen held the step ladder steady, and she heard him let out a long sigh.

"What's the sigh about?"

"Sorry, just looking at your beautiful figure from this vantage point and thinking about the future."

"I think you'd better lock up those thoughts for a couple more days, Mr. Morris."

"I'm trying, honest I am!"

After they hung the curtains they walked around the apartment making a list, then they sat on the couch discussing what was left to do for the wedding and the reception. When the list was complete, Jan turned to Allen. "Now I want to know, honestly, how you are dealing with Dad's death."

"You know, I did a lot of soul searching these last two days while I was at the ranch. I took some long walks around the property and stood at the mine shaft where we found him just about a year ago now. I came to the conclusion, it must have been his time to go. He had shown all of us what a changed man he was and I'm sure he did a lot of contemplating himself. He was allowed to live so we wouldn't remember him the dreadful way he was. I have to admit, it's been a lot easier to say goodbye, knowing how great he'd become. I'm going to miss him being a grandfather to our children. I will miss him during the holidays and I'll just miss him in my life. As Mom said, they've had their time together. Now it's time for us to carry on from here."

"How is she taking it?"

"She's a rock! She has the rest of her life planned out. She's going to sell the cattle and animals, keeping a couple of horses. She plans to stay up there for awhile; she's going to ask Barb if she would like to stay there with her. Eventually she plans on handing the ranch over to us if we want it and we'll go from there. How are you doing?"

"Like you said, I'm going to miss him, but I will always remember what a great man he was. Will it bother you to be at the cabin now that he's gone?"

"Having you with me, I think not! Speaking of the ranch, I have another surprise for you."

"What now?"

"Remember when I took you up that steep hill and told you it was my favorite view?"

"I'll never forget it since you were doing something illegal."

"What was illegal?"

Jan laughed, "Trespassing, you dufus!"

"Not when I own it."

Jan gasped, "What?"

"Honey, I bought that with my severance pay from the service."

"You mean we could build a home there someday?"

"Why do you think I took you up there? I wanted to get your reaction, and it was perfect."

"Well. Now that you've sprung another surprise on me, I'd better get over to Barb's and get ready to become the next Mrs. Morris. I'm going to be really busy tomorrow, so why don't we just plan on meeting together as I walk up the aisle?"

"You mean I can't stay with you tonight at Aunt Barb's?"

"Not a chance!" she said as she closed the door behind her.

CHAPTER FORTY FOUR
WE CAN STUFF IT WITH TOWELS

The next two days were a blur of activity. Everyone was going non-stop in their well planned directions. Jan went to bed at Aunt Barb's the night before her wedding thinking how everything had fallen into place in spite of the funeral. She was so grateful for her two mothers, Barb and her sister, Judy. They had done so much to help her. She was also grateful to her classmates who had stepped up and taken over the decorations.

She got up one more time to read over the list for tomorrow and came to the conclusion everything was in order. She returned to the bed, turned to her side and stared at the wall; suddenly she realized tomorrow night, she and Allen would be alone in their hotel room. She jumped out of bed and began pacing around the room.

I can't go through with this! How can we suddenly become intimate when we have learned to hold back for so long? What if I do something wrong? Maybe I can talk him into waiting for a few days. Great. Now I can't sleep. Oh, no. I'll have dark circles and bags under my eyes for the wedding. I think I'm driving myself crazy with my insignificant fears. Maybe I should try what I did the night before my speech. I'll get back to bed and do it.

Jan woke up with a start as the sun brightened her room. She went in to take her shower when she heard a knock on the door. "Who is it?"

"It's your sister, Judy."

"Come on in." she said as she threw a robe around her. "I was just getting into the shower. What's up?"

"It's your wedding day, that's what! No, actually I came to ask you what time the bridal shop opens so I can send Rick to pick up your wedding dress. Then I can give you my full attention."

"Sounds great. It opens at nine."

"Take your shower; I'll be back in a little bit. Oh, Aunt Barb said breakfast will be ready for the 'royal party' in 30 minutes."

Jan was kidding herself that she could eat. She nibbled on a piece of bacon while she twirled her fork around the eggs. Finally she said, "I'm going to pack my suitcase for tonight. Judy, would you go out to my car and get the white box from the back seat for me?"

"No, you're a big girl now, you can get your own box! Just kidding, little sister."

As Judy pushed her chair back, Jan heard Mandy's voice. "Knock, knock. Can I come in?"

"Come in the dining room, Mandy."

"Yes, your majesty, your lady-in-waiting is reporting for duty." Mandy quipped.

"Well, sit down, lady, and have some breakfast."

"I'm not about to turn down a free meal since I'm living alone now." Mandy said gleefully.

"Your hair's wet Miss Winston. I should put it in these new things I bought just to fix your hair. She opened a bag as she asked, "Miss Barb, do you mind if I do this at the table?"

"Not at all. Anything for the future Mrs. Morris! I'll hold your breakfast for you, Mandy."

"Thank you."

Mandy set to work with some kind of new devices, winding Jan's long hair precisely the way she wanted them to go.

"Would you like to tag along on our honeymoon so you can fix my hair every morning?"

"I'll bet Allen would love that. I'll just cuddle up between you."

"Mandy, I'm afraid the bed would break!"

"No problem. We'll put Allen on the couch and you can cuddle with me."

"I don't think I like where this is going."

The phone rang and Barb answered it. "Hello. No you can't talk to her or see her until she walks down the aisle! Okay, I'll ask her. He wants to know if Rick is coming over to go to the tux shop with him."

"Yes, after he brings me my wedding dress which he's on his way to pick up now."

"Did you hear that? Okay, bye."

Jan packed her bags. Mandy did her nails and makeup. Her dress was hanging in a plastic bag on the bedroom door. Everyone was fussing around Jan-between moms, sister, and bridesmaids, it was crazy. Mandy said, "You need to put on your dress now so I have plenty of time to do your hair before we leave for the church."

The moms took it out of the bag. They covered Jan's face with a paper bag so she wouldn't get her makeup on the dress. Jan heard someone let out a gasp as they pulled her dress on over her head. She pulled the bag off and looked down at her dress, screaming, "Oh no! It's huge! This isn't my dress! It can't be my dress. It doesn't even look like my dress. This is terrible!"

Her mother ran over to look at the name on the bag, and she said, "It's for a Winter's wedding. They must have given Rick the wrong dress."

Barb said, "Let me call the Bridal Shop and find out what's going on."

Jan stood there on the verge of tears, looking at her mom, and asked, "Mom, can you take it in?"

"Oh, honey, not only is it too big, it's also too long. We don't have the time necessary to fix it."

Mandy spoke up. "It's possible they gave your dress to the bride that had this dress, and she couldn't possibly fit in your dress. She's probably having a hissy fit also!"

Barb came running upstairs. "The store took my address and they are going to try to exchange the dresses. They'll deliver it; they feel terrible about the mistake!"

"So do I!" Jan said as she stepped out of the dress and sat down on the edge of the bed. Do you think they'll get it here in time? The wedding starts in one hour."

"Let me go ahead with your hair, and all you'll have to do is carefully slide into your dress," Mandy said softly.

"If it gets here in time," Jan said in a negative tone.

"Hey, it's no problem. If it doesn't, we'll stuff this dress with some towels and put you on stilts to walk down the aisle." Mandy's laughter brought some levity to the atmosphere.

Mandy worked on her hair, pinning her curls on the top of Jan's head and around the sides. Her hair was befitting a queen. She topped it off with her veil, and everyone let out superlatives of admiration. Barb came running up again and reported, "Okay, I called Allen to let him know why we might be a little late, and then the store called to say they retrieved your dress and the driver would be here in a few minutes."

Jan looked at the clock. "It takes 15 minutes to get to the church. The wedding is supposed to start in 20 minutes. Okay, we're going to be late, but we'll make the best of this."

Beverly said, "It's something to tell your kids about."

"You're right. Things couldn't possibly go smoothly at a wedding. There would be no funny stories to tell later." Judy added.

Mandy continued to do last-minute touch up on Jan's hair and makeup as they waited.

The doorbell rang; Barb took off like a NASCAR driver from the start line! As she came back up the stairs, she hollered, "This is it. It's your wedding dress and you'll never believe what they said!"

They decided to let her step into it so she wouldn't mess up her hair. Everyone helped her, then Jan turned to Aunt Barb. "What did they say?"

"They're returning half the price of the dress to make amends for the mistake."

Jan's mom said, "Wow. It was worth the wait."

By the time Jan was shuttled in and out of the car, she had no time to be nervous. When they walked her up to the front door of the church, her nervous system sprang into action, and she came close to disintegrating into miniscule pieces.

They were able to start ushering the mothers in exactly 20 minutes late. The groomsmen and bridesmaids made their entrance while Barb fussed with Jan's dress and veil. Jan's dad stood beaming at his little girl as he stood beside her. She took his arm as the wedding march began its familiar strain. Jan could see Allen's radiant smile directed toward her and was pleasantly surprised to see Pete standing beside Allen as she and her dad kept in perfect step to the music. Jan and her dad stood waiting as the minister asked who was giving the bride away. Her dad embellished the words a bit as he said, "With pride and pleasure I give my daughter to Allen Morris."

Allen took Jan's hand, feeling his tremors match her own. The minister gave a beautiful, meaningful talk about the significance of the marriage covenant, admonishing them to cleave to one another and no other. The emotions rose to new heights, as they exchanged their sacred vows.

Then the minister said, "You may kiss your bride."

Allen carefully lifted her veil, kissing her sweetly once. He pulled back, looking at her, and kissed her again. They turned as the minister announced, "Please welcome Mr. and Mrs. Allen and Janet Morris!"

They walked out amidst smiles and clapping. They were ushered out by the photographer and the formal picture taking commenced. Forty-five minutes later, they walked into the reception hall. Jan was thrilled to see the decorations which the girls did. They were more elegant then she expected. They assembled into a receiving line. Many well wishers came through, quite a few offering their condolences to Carmela and Allen. It was a difficult reminder that Frank wasn't there. They were finally allowed to sit down and someone placed a plate of food in front of each of them. They were able to mix in a bite or two as people continued to come up and talk to them. Rick came up behind them and said, "I don't see any champagne available to make the toast."

Allen explained, "Rick, we're just serving apple juice mixed with 7-up for the toast."

"What? Well, I'll just run out and get a few bottles of bubbly to serve those who want it."

Jan decided to step in. "No you won't Rick, this church doesn't allow any alcohol in their building or on the grounds, so you'll have to make do with the juice."

"What kind of stupid church is this? And it's your wedding. Everyone serves alcohol for the toast!"

Jan had not seen this side of Rick before, he was usually so level-headed. She noticed from the corner of her eye, her sister approaching. Judy quietly said, "Rick, leave it alone. It's not your wedding, and you can handle one reception without alcohol, okay?"

"This is ridiculous," he muttered as he walked away with Judy pulling on his arm.

Jan turned to Allen. "Well, that was fun."

Suddenly Jan's dad stepped up to the microphone. "May I have your attention, please?" Jan groaned as she knew how verbal her dad could be. "Everyone quiet, please." Slowly the murmuring subsided. "Everyone needs to get a glass from the table so we can make a toast, please." Some moved around to get his or her juice and when everyone was quiet again, her dad continued. "Ladies and gentlemen, I propose a toast to the new Mr. and Mrs. Morris; may your lives together continue to develop and nurture the profound love you feel towards one another at this moment. May you support each other throughout your marriage and unite your love to bring us lots of grandchildren!"

Pete, who stood in as Allen's best man, came over to the mic. "I'd like to say a few words to the happy couple. I've known the handsome groom for most of my life and all I can say to you, Allen, is that you are sure one lucky man!"

Jan's dad then announced, "Looks like the band is ready, so the bride and groom will approach the dance floor to display the real reason they want to be together for the rest of their lives. Jan and Allen approached the dance floor; her train had been conveniently hooked up to her dress so she was free to dance. "Please welcome Allen and Janet dancing to their love song."

A male singer stepped up to the microphone and the band started playing "The Twelfth of Never." Allen took Janet in his arms and began moving her around the floor in a smooth waltz. He easily maneuvered her into several twirls and back again as they continued throughout the meaningful song. When the band stopped playing, people cheered, but they only had eyes for each other. Allen kissed her and said, "You mean everything to me. You're my world, the love of my life." He kissed her one more time.

Jan's dad came back to the microphone. "Just a little tidbit about this happy couple. They were each taught to dance at a very early age. Yet they dated for almost two years without knowing how they both loved to dance. Can you see why they were brought together?"

The crowd gave them another round of applause.

Suddenly the band leader brought them back to reality as he announced the parents' dance. Allen took his mother in his arms, and Jan's dad did the same with his daughter. He asked "Is my little girl happy?"

"More like ecstatic!"

"He's a good man, honey. I'm very happy with your choice."

"Dad, you'll have to dance with me twice so Allen can dance with his new mother-in-law."

"Oh, really. And who might she be? I'd better watch them so I can cut in and hold her in my arms next."

"I think she'd like that Daddy."

The dancing continued for close to two hours until Judy came up to them and said, "It's time to cut the cake, kids. The lions are ready to pounce if they don't get their dessert!"

They cut the cake and each fed the other a small bite and then continued to feed each other the rest of the piece of cake. Jan said, "Thank you for not smearing the cake on me."

"Now why would I want to do that to the most beautiful face in the world? Besides, it would give the impression I have no respect for you, wouldn't it?"

"When I think about it, I suppose it would. Now you have the privilege of taking off my garter, Mr. Morris."

"Oh, now I will certainly enjoy doing that, Mrs. Morris!"

They threw the garter and her flowers. It wasn't completely coincidental when Rob caught the garter and Mandy retrieved the flowers.

They danced a couple more dances, then Judy sent them off to change clothes. Mandy accompanied Jan so she could touch up her makeup. She was stunning in her outfit, and Allen changed to dress slacks, a white shirt and tie with a sport jacket.

Everyone lined the walkway and threw rice at them as they ran through. The car had cans and balloons attached and a sign in the back that said "Just Married!"

They waved goodbye and drove away to begin their life together as a married couple.

CHAPTER FORTY FIVE
THE OUTHOUSE

As they drove towards their hotel, Allen said, "Are you hungry?"

"I'm starved."

"I made a reservation at the same restaurant where I proposed. Are you alright with that?"

"I'd love it. What time is it anyway?"

"Half passed kissing time. Time to kiss again!"

"Allen, patience."

"Okay, it's almost seven o'clock."

Jan had a hot roast beef sandwich, and Allen had a steak.

"I thought I was hungry, but I can barely eat even half my sandwich."

"That's how you always eat, Pumpkin. I'll bet you could go for a hot fudge sundae though."

"You know me so well. Could we share one?"

"Absolutely."

Allen ordered, then he moved over beside her to share the sundae. As he slid in next to her he said, "You seem distracted and nervous, Jan. Can I help?'

"Not really, I'm just trying to prepare myself, sweetheart."

"Prepare yourself for what?"

Jan began to flush. "You know. I can't talk about it in public."

"Maybe we need to talk when we get to our room, okay?"

Mentioning the room made her want to jump up and run away, but was saved by the sundae.

They fed it to each other, giggling as Allen kissed off whipped cream that landed on her lips. "People are going to think we're some kind of freaks, Allen."

"You know what?"

"What?"

"I don't care what other people think!"

Jan put the spoon down and said, "I can't eat another bite."

"Okay, let me get the bill and we'll go to the hotel."

Jan was really struggling with her nerves at the mention of the hotel.

They drove to it, took their suitcases out and let the valet park the car. They walked up to the desk and Allen said, "We have reservations for the bridal suite. The name is Morris."

"Yes, sir. Let me just check. Ah, yes, Here it is. Would you like to settle the bill when you leave in the morning?"

"Yes, that would be fine."

The clerk handed Allen a key as he said, with a hint of a grin, "Do enjoy your stay in our hotel. Check out time is 12 noon."

They started for the elevator when Jan stopped. "Allen, when we get in our room, I really do want to talk to you."

"Sure Pumpkin, as long as it doesn't take all night."

They entered an empty elevator, and as the door closed, Jan slid close to him. "This is the first time I've been in an elevator since you know when."

Without saying a word, Allen put his arms around her in a loving embrace and kissed her like he'd never kissed her before.

Jan reciprocated with all her heart, body and soul as she experienced a tingling sensation never felt before. She wanted to feel it more.

They entered the room. Allen put the bags down and asked her what she wanted to talk about.

She moved closer to him. "I was going to talk about some of my fears regarding intimacy, but after that elevator kiss, I don't think it's necessary. All you have to do is kiss me that way again."

"With pleasure, Mrs. Morris!"

***

It was about two in the morning, and the amorous couple was laughing at their shared nervousness of a few hours earlier. They sat together in an enormous heart shaped bath tub taking a bubble bath. As they soaked, they were drinking in the marvelous event they had just shared together. It was a whole new world opening up in their relationship.

Allen said, "I could never have imagined in a million years how beautiful you are and how deeply I love you."

Jan slid close and said, "I hope you can feel the tremendous emotions I'm experiencing for you now. I never imagined that love could be so all consuming."

"I know exactly what you mean. I just want to hold you and continue this feeling for the rest of our lives together."

"I believe that's part of the plan, is it not?"

"Yes, Pumpkin, I'm sure it is."

They laughed together in the intimacy of this special night, helping each other dry off, looking forward to many such moments shared together.

* * *

As Jan awoke wrapped in the arms of her husband, she knew there couldn't be another person on earth feeling more joy than she did at this moment. She turned over to face him as he started to awaken. "Good morning, Pumpkin."

"Good morning, sweetheart. Can you see what time it is?"

"Now what do you want to know the time for? We're on our honeymoon, darling!"

"Didn't you hear the clerk say we had to check out by noon? And we have a 4 or 5 hour drive to the cabin, right?"

"Okay, its nine thirty, and we have plenty of time for . . ."

She cuddled in closer as she giggled, "Time for what?"

He answered with a long, wonderful kiss, and she knew exactly what they had time for.

* * *

As they drove the dirt road leading to the cabin, Jan was amazed at the beauty surrounding them. They were on the edge of a small, secluded valley with a river winding its way through it. They crested a small hill, and she could see the green roof of the cabin. They pulled up beside it, and she didn't wait for Allen to open the car door before she jumped out. Jan could smell the pine trees and the freshness of the air with a bit of a nip to it. There were huge outcroppings of granite rocks, bushes and spring flowers of lavender, yellow and deep rose dotting the steep hill in back of the cabin. She ran down into the meadow to the river, leaning down to dip her fingers in the water. The ice-cold water from the spring snow melt shocked her momentarily, as she quickly withdrew her hand. There were still patches of snow isolated in areas of shade. She turned to go back, and Allen was quietly standing behind her drinking in her enthusiasm with a sweet grin on his face.

"Allen, this is beautiful. I don't ever want to leave this place. I love it here!"

"You haven't seen the inside of the cabin yet. Or for that matter, the outhouse!"

"Well, what are we waiting for. Let's go."

As they walked back to the cabin, Allen felt uneasy about the inside as he said, "Janet, remember how I told you the cabin is very primitive, and since my folks were unable to come up to clean things before we arrived as they intended, it has sat all winter gathering dirt."

"So. We'll just have to clean it right?"

They walked up the steps that were made from old logs to the front porch that extended the length of the cabin. Allen explained, "We have to open the wood shutters first. They've been closed to protect the windows from the snow. I'll show you how to do it, and then I can get the ladder to open the higher ones on the side of the cabin, okay?"

The shutters had simple locks, making them easy to open. When she finished the front, Jan went around to the back to do the same. As she passed Allen on the ladder, she asked, "Can I help you with that?"

"I don't think two of us can fit on this ladder, sweetheart."

"I know. It was fun to ask."

While in the back, Jan saw the outhouse a short distance behind the cabin at the end of a narrow little path. She ventured up to take a look, and even though she'd never seen one before, she mused that it was really quite nice. She opened the nicely varnished toilet seat cover to look inside and jumped back from the offensive odor and flies that emerged! *Yes, I have to agree, it is quite primitive! But I'll get used to it (I hope)!*

Allen came around the corner just as she was starting down the path. "Did you use it?"

"No, I just looked inside."

"Good, because I have to treat it with lye and fly spray."

"Will the lye get rid of the odor?"

"I guess, until someone poops in it."

"Oh, honey, did you have to tell me that?"

"No, just wanted to see your reaction."

When they entered the inside of the cabin, it was decorated just the way a mountain cabin should be. Mom had made adorable red and green curtains for the windows, covers for the beds with lots of throw pillows and cute knickknacks to make it homey. Allen took her to a ladder in the back leading to a loft with three more beds. While they were in the loft, Allen took the cover off one of the beds, drawing her down on top of the blanket. He kissed her, and then kissed her again, and before they knew it they plunged into that special sacred union between husband and wife.

After cleaning the cabin together, they cooked dinner on the antique wood stove in the kitchen. As darkness approached, they sat cuddled in each other's arms on the front porch. Allen taught Jan how to light the kerosene lanterns, and as the evening progressed, the temperature dropped remarkably, forcing them inside to play double solitaire by the light of a lantern. The kitchen stove kept the cabin warm until the wood burned down leading them to the refuge of the warm covers in the downstairs bed. As they cuddled together, it seemed nothing could destroy this rapturous moment. Their joy was so complete; it felt like it could last forever.

While laying there in the dark, Jan asked, "Have you ever been frightened in the dark of night in this perfect mountain paradise?"

"No, except when a wild animal decides to join us inside the cabin."

Jan jumped. "What kind of animals?"

"Big, huge mountain mice, raccoons, squirrels and big black bears. Grrrrrr." he said as he nuzzled his nose in her neck.

"Allen, you're scaring me!"

"Why? You know I'll protect you with my 'superman' strength."

They went off to sleep giggling like a couple of young school kids.

If they only knew what tomorrow would bring, they'd abandon ship immediately and run for cover.

CHAPTER FORTY SIX
A NIGHTMARE RELIVED

Jan and Allen awakened early with the morning sun welcoming them to another stupendous day. "Pumpkin, you stay under the covers while I light the fire in the stove and warm it up in here."

"What a great idea," she said as she snuggled into the covers.

"In fact, I'll even fix some breakfast for you while I'm up." Allen kissed her cheek as he reached around to pull himself up.

"You are the best husband in the whole wide world. Now will you step outside in the cold and go potty for me while you're at it?"

"I would if I could, but if you don't get around, I'll have breakfast all by myself."

"You won't serve me in bed?" Jan asked while she turned over to sit up on the side of the bed.

"Not at the cabin. That's reserved for birthdays and Mother's Day. Well maybe when you're sick."

"You're no fun at all." Jan put her slippers and robe on, forcing herself out in the cold. In spite of the immediate chill, she stood outside the door and drank in the awakening of morning-the pungent smells of pine, a wisp of the smoke as the fire came to life in the old wood stove, chipmunks and birds making known their territorial boundaries. What a fantastic place to celebrate the newness of their lives together. A subtle breeze awakened her senses to the drop in temperature as she headed up the little hill.

Going potty in an "outhouse" was a new experience for Janet, but it was all a part of their "back to nature" experience, and after all they were struggling college students who couldn't afford a luxury honeymoon. *Maybe someday* Jan sighed.

While emptying her bladder, she thought she heard voices. She called out, "Sweetheart, is that you?"

She heard nothing, so she figured it must have been the wind blowing through the pine trees. She reached to flush the toilet then realized there was no toilet to flush! She giggled to herself as she pulled her pajama bottoms up and tied her robe around her waist. She pushed open the outhouse door, stepping carefully onto the path. She suddenly felt something behind her. Before she could react, an arm went roughly around her waist, lifting her feet off the ground as a growling voice said, "Just take it easy sister and you won't get hurt."

She started to scream, and his other hand went forcefully over her mouth. "Shut up or my brother will blow your boyfriend's head off!"

In her terror, she wanted to call to Allen, knowing the men were headed inside the cabin. Above his filthy hand she could barely see another man sneaking up behind Allen. She tried to warn him, but her sounds were muffled by his hand.

Allen had heard the back door open and he was about to greet Jan, just as an arm went around his neck and a gun was forced into his back. He heard a raspy deep voice at his ear. "If you move, I'll shoot you dead, and then we'll have our way with the pretty little thing in my brother's arms."

Allen almost dropped to his knees as he realized who had slammed themselves back into his world. The brothers who a year ago left his father to die at the bottom of a mine shaft.

Peter Savio, the sheriff had told Allen several law enforcement agencies were going to try to flush them out from the mountains above the cabin. Were they on the run again?

Allen was forced to a chair and commanded to sit down, as the other brother roughly pulled Jan on the bed with a knife to her throat. The one behind Allen said, "If you make a move, my brother will slice her throat wide open!" He reached to tie Allen's hands behind the chair.

Coming around in front of Allen, he looked at him slowly, walked from side to side, placing his free hand on his chin as he studied Allen and said, "I know you from somewhere."

"Hey bro, the only place you know anyone is from jail," said the brother holding Jan hostage, snickering at his own bad joke.

"Wait a minute, you look so familiar. It's coming to me. You were a teenager. Yeah, a teenager at your dad's hearing. You're the son of Frank Morris!"

"No way, bro. Are you fibbing me?" He grabbed Jan's chin, turning her face toward him. "Hey little princess, what's your boyfriend's name?"

Jan defiantly answered, "I won't tell you."

"Hey, do you want my brother to put a bullet through his brain right now? Tell us what his name is girly!"

"Morris, Allen Morris."

"Well, howdy do and dandy, we got us Frank's son and his little playmate."

Allen was quietly evaluating their circumstances; formulating a plan of action. Jan wished she knew what he planned so she could be a part of it.

"Hey there, Allen old boy, this calls for a celebration. Got any whiskey hidden around this shack?" The brother waved the gun in front of Allen.

Allen shook his head no.

"Hey Bro, we still have a bottle in our backpack. Want me to go get it?"

"No, you keep the knife close to her throat. I'll get the bottle."

Jan was roughly pushed over while he maneuvered to get a better hold with his arm around her waist. He took the sharp point of the knife and pushed her robe aside at the neck. "Watch ya got under there, sweetie?"

Jan tried to pull away, looking at Allen in dismay.

"If you lay one hand on her, I will personally track you down and rip your eyeballs out!"

"Oh, ho ho! I'm shaken in my boots, little boyfriend." He said as he let out a raucous laugh, revealing brown spikes where his teeth should have been.

Jan barely recognized Allen, as he displayed a look in his eyes that terrified even her.

Just then the brother slammed through the door. "Okay, let's have a party, bro," he said as he took a swig out of a half-full bottle.

Allen hoped they'd get drunk to give him an advantage in judgment. His biggest concern in the meantime was their lusting over his precious Janet.

They took turns at their personal liquor store until the bottle was empty. Then they turned their attention towards Janet.

"Hey cutey, wouldn't you like to have a little fun? We've been without a women for over a year now. Don't ya want to help a couple of starving guys out?" He spoke into her ear as she backed away cringing.

One of them tried to kiss her while she turned her head back and forth. They hadn't tied her, thinking she was so tiny she didn't pose any threat. One brother handed the weapons to the other saying, "I'm going first, then you can have her; you watch the big man over there, shoot him if she fights me!"

He turned towards her, and as he tried to pull her pajama bottoms down, Jan flew into an orbit of her past memory. This propelled her into a sphere above her own body. She felt emboldened by an army of silent warrior angels that filled her with strength beyond her normal capacity. She suddenly went completely wild. She fought like a Ninja Warrior, scratching, biting, kicking and wriggling away with every bit of empowered strength within her.

"Whoa there, girl, you're a lively one. This is going to be fun."

The other brother came over to hold her down and that's when Allen made his move.

He'd been slowly working at the knots clumsily done in a hurry and pulled his arms free. He picked up the chair and swung around with it, knocking it over the head of one of them, sending the gun and knife slithering across the cabin. As the brother splattered to the floor, the other tried to pull up his pants, and Allen cold cocked him with a powerful right to his jaw!

Just then both doors flew open and law enforcement officers filled the cabin. Allen jumped to wrap Jan in his arms and help her maintain her modesty.

Peter Savio walked up saying, "Looks to me like you did our job for us, Allen. When we found their camp hastily abandoned, I had a hunch they might make it down to your cabin. We came as quickly as we could. I'm really sorry, Allen. This shouldn't have happened to you and Janet. I feel so responsible."

The bloody brothers were handcuffed and taken away. Pete turned to Janet and Allen asking, "Are either of you hurt in any way? Before they could answer, he turned to Jan with a fierce look of dismay. "Janet, did they get to you?"

Allen laughed, "Let me tell you, Pete, my little bride is a ferocious little fighter when it comes to someone invading her sacred space. Because of her, it gave me the chance to take them down. Remind me never to get on her bad side. But I'm sure glad you arrived when you did. I hope you can put them away for as long as we both walk on this earth. They're nothing but bad news."

"You have no idea how happy I am to be able to add to their attempted murder charges, kidnapping and attempted rape! We're going to lock them up and forget they ever existed. Will you be willing to testify in court against them?" Pete asked, looking at both of them.

Jan spoke first. "I can hardly wait!"

"Count me in as well, Pete."

"Alright, we will leave you two alone to enjoy the rest of your honeymoon; you sure you're both okay? I can leave a couple of my deputies around to watch the place."

Allen smiled, "As long as I have Janet here to protect me, we don't need any babysitters."

"We'll be fine, Pete," Jan said emphatically.

"Couldn't have said it better myself," Allen reiterated.

"Good luck to you kids. Frank would be real proud of you right now. Too bad he had to die so unexpectedly. He could have been a part of rounding them up."

"Did you find their camp at Peep Site?"

"Yeah, it was a ways below it, but they must have seen us coming, and that's how they landed down here. I'm really sorry we didn't get here sooner, Allen."

"No problem. My little sweetheart here was in full control before I finished them off."

The sheriff laughed as he went out the door, and Allen and Jan waved as he drove off.

When they were back in the cabin, Allen took Jan in his arms, saying, "I'm so sorry you had to experience such a horrible thing, Pumpkin. Are you sure you're alright?"

"I'm fine, really. Just feel terribly dirty where they had their slimy hands on me. I wish I could take a hot shower."

"You can, sweetheart. Let me get the hot water going on the stove."

"You're kidding me. Where's the shower?"

"Come here," he took her behind the kitchen. "Now look up."

Jan looked up and saw a large round sturdy canvas bag hanging beside the ladder to the loft. "Why didn't I notice this before?"

"Because you only had eyes for me."

"You're absolutely right," she said as she hugged him. "Okay, now tell me how I do this."

"As soon as the water heats up, I'll explain everything. You know what, I smell bacon."

"We never ate breakfast, did we? And now it's probably cooking again on top of the stove."

"Madam, would you care for a bit of well-cooked breakfast?"

"Lead the way, chef."

They sat down to some overdone eggs and bacon when Jan asked, "What do we have planned for dinner?"

"I'm going to teach you the fine art of Dutch oven cooking in the fire pit."

"That sounds fascinating. Will that lesson come after my shower?"

"Yes indeed it will. I believe the water is hot so please go and take off your clothes."

"Excuse me?"

"Oh, honey, does that bother you after what just happened?"

"As long as you're sure they are long gone, I think I'll be okay with that."

"It's just you, me and the chickens," Allen said as he took Jan in his arms to give her a reassuring hug.

Jan felt so much better after her shower but disappointed Allen couldn't join her because he had to stand on the stairs and fill the bag with water. It was still fun. She kept sprinkling him with water until he was almost as wet as she was.

Once they cleaned up the cabin, put the meat and vegetables in the kettle and smothered it with red hot coals in the outdoor fire pit, they went for a long walk climbing up on top of some granite rocks. They began to talk intimately about the episode of the morning.

"Jan, you don't seem to be upset about it. Do you realize what they had intended to do to you?"

"Yes, I do, and all I could think about was preventing it. I guess because of my previous experience, I felt a deep seething anger towards them and used it to fight the only way I knew how."

"Honey, you fought like an animal. Where did that come from?"

"Somewhere deep, deep inside. Or, sort of somewhere else."

"What do you mean?"

"Well, I don't want you to think I'm crazy or weird, but something happened to me that I don't know how to explain."

"Honey, you know you can tell me anything."

"I know, but this is really far out. I felt like I was given some additional help from some angels or something. I know I don't have that kind of strength on my own, even with the adrenalin pumping." Jan looked at Allen as he sat up straight giving her a look of astonishment. Jan smiled reassuringly, "I know what you're thinking, and I'm surprised at it myself."

"Janet Morris, you never cease to amaze me. I keep seeing new layers of your inner self and I feel overwhelmed by what is revealed about you." He enveloped her in his arms and said, "I'll admit, when I thought I was going to witness such an act on my wife, I was overcome by an urge to murder both of them!"

"Well, I'm certainly glad it didn't come to that. As my mother often says, 'All's well that ends well'."

"You know, Jan, I've never been so completely taken off guard. It was so foreign to my memories of the cabin. We have never had any bad thing happen here, except the time a bear got in during the winter and messed things up."

"There are bears up here?"

"Of course, Pumpkin! Lions and tigers and bears!"

She got up and said, "I'll bet I can beat you back to the cabin."

"I'll just bet you can't."

They were breathless as they returned, flopping down on the bed to catch their breath and Allen turned to look at Jan saying, "Now why did you have to go and do that?"

"Do what?"

"Take off your clothes in front of me this morning and now lay down beside me."

"Are you saying I'm irresistible?"

He brought her into an embrace, "Yes, yes, you certainly are!"

* * *

They sat outside at the campfire roasting marshmallows after enjoying a fantastic dinner. It was starting to get dark when Jan said she would really prefer to be inside with the doors locked after dark.

"Are you frightened because of this morning?"

"Probably. I didn't feel this way yesterday. The dark makes me feel like something may be out there I can't see."

"I guarantee there's nothing to be afraid of. Well, maybe a big mountain lion!" He said as he jumped grabbing her in his arms, lifting her up to carry her into the cabin while holding her close in his embrace.

"See, I feel much better inside with the curtains closed, the doors locked and the lanterns on."

"So, it has nothing to do with my being here to protect you?"

"Heck no. You look just like the lion that carried me into the cabin."

"And that same lion just might attack you at any given moment."

"Is that a promise?"

"You bet it is my darling."

"Okay, now you've scared me; you're going with me to the outhouse so I can go potty."

"That sounds like a delightful idea. I'll get the flashlight."

* * *

Jan and Allen took long hikes nearly every day, high above the cabin for spectacular views. They investigated an abandoned mine shaft and drove to a ghost town. Each knew that their fantasy world would come to an end, and they would be facing the reality of work, school, study and keeping ahead of bills. For now their lives had started with the magic of knowing one another in such a way that brought a closeness that would endure the test of time. The memory of that dark morning faded away with each minute spent together exploring their deep and abiding love.

Driving home they felt almost giddy knowing they could face anything together and looked forward to the next chapters of their lives.

EPILOGUE

Janet and Allen settled down to a busy routine and often sustained each other in their individual endeavors to progress in their pursuits. Jan was dedicated to the practice of nursing at Watkins Medical Center and diligently extended herself to receive promotions that would allow her to make suggestions for change.

Allen continued work at the gas station while pursuing his education in dentistry.

By now Allen had confided the secrets he withheld before their marriage about the funds from his father. They now had dreams of eventually building their final home on top of their mountain.

They continued to have a close relationship with Mandy and Rob who had a very private small wedding a few months after theirs. Kim and her fiancé were busy making plans for an elaborate ceremony. The three nurses remained close on and off duty, supporting each other as best friends. Cindy and Dave remained in the picture but had distanced themselves due to differences in life style. They remained friends, and Cindy often confided in Jan.

An atmosphere of change permeated through the sixties and seventies, allowing registered nurses to come into their own, removing the shackles of the Dark Ages. It was an exciting time for these new, energetic nurses determined to make a difference in the lives of their patients and in their chosen profession.

Many new experiences came about at the medical center while Jan and Allen's personal lives were often plagued by the trials and tribulations which will be encountered in the sequel that follows.

www.ingramcontent.com/pod-product-compliance
Lightning Source LLC
Chambersburg PA
CBHW081234180526
45171CB00005B/426